'Childhood' in 'Crisis'?

'Childhood' in 'Crisis'?

Edited by

Phil Scraton

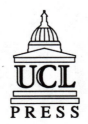

UCL

PRESS

First published in 1997 by UCL Press

UCL Press Limited
1 Gunpowder Square
London EC4A 3DE
UK

and

1900 Frost Road, Suite 101
Bristol
Pennsylvania 19007-1598
USA

The name University College London (UCL) is a registered trade mark Used by
UCL Press with the consent of the owner.

British Library Cataloguing-in-Publication Data
A catalogue record for this book is available from the British Library.

Library of Congress Cataloging-in-Publication Data are available

ISBNs: 1-85728-788-6 (HB)
       1-85728-789-4 (PB)

Typeset in 10/12pt Times
by Best-set Typesetter Ltd, Hong Kong

Printed by SRP Ltd, Exeter

Contents

Contents

Preface

Throughout the 1990s widely-proclaimed assumptions about the demise of childhood, the ill-discipline of children and the lawlessness of youth have dominated popular discourses and political reaction. Widespread condemnation of the erosion of family life and the decline of school standards as the central institutions of children's socialization, has fuelled adult indignation and claims of a 'lost generation' of young people. A litany of the deviants has been constructed providing evidence that the social and moral fabric of British society is collapsing, infected at its childhood foundations. The streets, it is argued, are inhabited by drug users, runaways, joyriders and persistent young offenders. Schools suffer the excesses of bullies, truants and disruptive pupils. Families have become 'dismembered', replaced by lone mothers, characterized by absent fathers. Whatever the broader political–economic context, the growing divide between conspicuous, affluent consumerism and below-the-breadline existence, the judgmental finger of marginalization and exclusion points at pathological individuals and degenerate communities. 'Childhood' is in 'crisis', children lack appropriate discipline, parental control or professional guidance. The political message, broadly consensual across the main parties, is that *we* (meaning the collective of responsible adulthood) have become too soft, too understanding and too tolerant. Thatcher's 1980s 'return to Victorian values' was superseded by Major's 'back to basics' initiative, his rallying call in the war on 'yob culture'. Not to be overshadowed, New Labour's Tony Blair called for an awakening of the 'sleeping conscience of the country' to guard against the potential of 'moral chaos which engulfs us all'.

The catalyst for this outpouring of adult condemnation, directed remorselessly against contemporary childhood, was the killing in February 1993 of a young child, James Bulger, and the subsequent arrest and conviction of two 10-year-old children. It came hard on the heels of moral panics over escalating crime, no-go areas and the 'rising underclass'. It was portrayed as the extreme end of a developing continuum of children's aberrant and criminal behaviour, the inevitable outcome of the breakdown of parental and community discipline. Although a rare and exceptional event, the circumstances of James Bulger's death and the violence of the two boys gave rise to a prolonged and generalized condemnation of children, families and communities. The intensity, style and content of adult reaction was unprecedented. While such an abduction and violent killing defies immediate comprehension, the process of pathologization of the two boys was compounded by the trial judge's description of their act as one of 'unparalleled evil'. It was a sentiment echoed throughout the media which emphasized the subjugation of 'innocence' and repeatedly portrayed the event as representative of the potential for evil in all children. Their crime was accentuated precisely because they were children. This premise underpinned much of the comment on the case demonstrating the ease with which adults, be they parents, politicians, journalists, judges, or professional experts, define and determine the personalities and actions of children. At the centre of the subsequent, much-publicized debates has remained the persistent assumption that childhood innocence requires protection from the forces of evil which lie dormant, but waiting to be triggered, in the minds and chemistry of a pathological minority. And so the definers become the protectors, determining 'what is best' for society's children, exactly what and when they need to know and experience. Innocence becomes synonymous with *näiveté* and, inevitably, *näiveté* constitutes the foundation of ignorance. Adults become the judges and keepers of the 'best interests' of the child.

Perhaps more than any other decade, the 1990s has been characterized, by open displays of adult indignation, as the decade which marks the end of childhood innocence. This theme, covering crime, deviance, sex, sexuality, school, families, magazines, television, videos – the list is endless – has been obsessive. Police concerns about 'persistent young offenders', for example, provoked journalists into chasing after the most lurid and exaggerated stories of children's involvement in crime. Masked children, possibly armed, stared through the eye-holes of balaclavas from the pages of hyped feature articles while television documentaries used night-sights on their cameras to relay the 'nastiest' behaviour from the 'worst' estates. A 'rat-boy', supposedly living rough among the ventilation shafts and cellars of flats and houses, was revealed to be operating in the North-East. Each sweep search for the child with the highest number of offences, recorded or not, threw up fresh examples of the uncontrollable and the uncontainable. 'Is This the Worst Child in Britain?' demanded headlines as yet another excessively 'naughty' child was presented by the press to the nation. This led to a parade of children and young people expelled from school whose parents demanded their reinstatement. Clearly not all such cases were fabricated or even exaggerated but what this exceptional media concentration achieved was an over-generalization and misrepresentation of the issues. When pressed for numbers of 'persistent young offenders', for example, the Home Office could only produce a figure slightly over 100. Yet the moral panic was already fully amplified.

John Major, along with the spokespeople for other parties, used his prime ministerial weight to urge the nation to 'condemn a little more' and 'understand a little less'. At the very moment when informed analysis and understanding of the complexities was most needed, the political agenda was set to condemn, demonize and punish. Certainly, little attention was given to understanding. While divided on so much else, the Conservative Party united around spurious academic analyses of the growing *'underclass'*, typified by lone mothers, ill-disciplined children, 'fatherless communities', spiralling crime, indiscriminate violence, unteachable pupils and low moral standards. This was presented as the rising spectre of the *dangerous classes* – nineteenth century revisited occupied by Fagin's thieves, idlers and unemployables. Unexpectedly this well-worn line of right-wing rhetoric drew considered support from self-styled 'ethical socialists' who linked the decline of the family and the absence of fathers to the breakdown of working-class communities and the creation of irresponsible youth. Again, a political consensus prevailed revealing a broad acceptance of the decline of academic, social and moral standards among children and young people. Significantly, the 'crisis' in 'childhood' was no longer presented as uni-dimensional. It was not restricted to anti-social behaviour or criminal acts but was inclusive of a range of social experience. The primary, formal locations of children's socialization – the family and the school – became the principal targets of those who talked up the *'crisis'*, those who sought institutional causation and tangible scapegoats.

Inevitably, these aggressive and highly-charged debates have not been without consequences. With little reference to history, the assumption has been that the 'crisis' is unique, demanding immediate and strong intervention. In keeping with a broader agenda of social authoritarianism, it has resulted in a broad range of legislative and policy reform directed towards its resolution. What follows is a critical examination of the dynamics behind the political debate and its consequences for policy. Part One provides the central historical and theoretical frameworks and considers the expansive media coverage and popular discourse which collectively contextualize legal and policy responses. In developing the work it was considered appropriate to review the conceptualization of children and social construction of childhood from eighteenth century roots through to nineteenth century manifestations. Given what is introduced above, it is salutary to revisit nineteenth century bourgeois perceptions and fears relating to political sedition and subversion, morality panics generated by deeply-held assumptions about corruption and contagion, and the emergence of Victorian philanthropy as a principal influence in the construction of contemporary childhood. Important here is the development of institutions and organizations specifically oriented towards children and their paradoxical fusion of care, control and contempt. From these institutional and policy foundations the review moves on to overview the key twentieth century policy developments, a primary focus being the period of post-1945 reconstruction including the development of the Welfare State and the consolidation of specialized child-care policies, professions and services.

What this historical overview demonstrates is the dynamic relationships between societal change, state intervention, legal definition, social policy and contrasting theories of childhood. In Part One the dominant theoretical paradigms (conservatism, liberalism and structural functionalism) are outlined, contrasted and critiqued. This is followed by a consideration of the imperatives of political–economic analyses and the contribution of critical perspectives which focus on the power relations underpinning the social and political construction of childhood and child–adult relations. Significant here has been, and remains, the care v. control debate particularly in terms of the determining contexts and structural relations of class, gender, sexuality and 'race'. In developing a critical analysis of power relations which determine definitions of, and access to, rights for children and young people there is the vexed question of the contrasting conceptualization of *inherent vulnerability* and *structural vulnerability*.

From this historical and theoretical overview and critique there follows a critical examination of contemporary popular discourse and media coverage of 'childhood'. The discussion of the influence of the media as '*powerful definers*' or gatekeepers, particularly relating to children and young people as social deviants or offenders, develops much of that previously mentioned. The profound contradictions between portrayals and representations of children as vulnerable innocents in need of protection and the media images of an ascendant 'yob culture' requiring strict discipline, constant surveillance and harsh punishment has provided popular legitimation for authoritarian interventions. Clearly the James Bulger case was a critical point in the intensification of the 'moral panic' around children and crime. It unleashed an unprecedented level of media attention on a global scale which was refocused on *childhood* in general terms. The style, content and over-generalization of this coverage requires consideration alongside that which has prevailed around much more common crimes involving children: as victims of physical and sexual abuse perpetrated by adults. What this analysis examines is the contradiction evident between the concerned rhetoric of care and the regulatory reality of control within the context of an increasingly divided society.

Part Two of the book considers the principal sites of the debate over childhood and the statutory and non-statutory policy responses and agency interventions. It focuses on the family, sexuality, schooling, youth justice and mental health developing a detailed historical and contemporary account of the significant issues within each of these distinct but related areas. As noted above, society's health and well-being is represented consistently as being bound inextricably to the social arrangements of the nuclear family within an extended and caring context. In this idealized model children are brought up in households of two, preferably married, parents alongside their siblings. They are introduced to their parents' families through the extended network of grandparents and other significant relatives. It is this core together with the broader familial network which, according to the moral–political rhetoric of the New Right and ethical socialists alike, has disintegrated. What is significant here is a critical appraisal of the family, a cultural and historical creation, as the primary, unidimensional context for child-rearing. Central to this is the idealization of the family which masks the significance and force, physical and ideological, of power relations based on age and gender. The family remains pivotal to much British social policy and legislation, defining and delimiting relationships and responsibilities. It is also deeply significant in the interventions of child agencies and their professionals. While much has been made of the advances of children's rights through national legislation and international conventions, there is a clear need to assess real progress against the lived experiences of children and young people. This broader debate raises the often unpalatable but crucial question for young people of the relevance of idealized portrayals of the 'functional family' to their lives.

One of the most volatile debates concerning young people, bringing with it significant changes in legislation and policy, has centred on sex, sexuality and access to reliable information. The chapter on sexuality considers the traditional child development emphasis which assumes that at some point, directly related to biological growth, young people experience a transition which equips them, via guidance, to make appropriate judgments about sexual relations. Connected to this have been the moral–philosophical debates which construct 'appropriate' sexual behaviour based on an assumed relationship between biology, morality and pleasure and the medico–legal discourses about nature, 'normality' and regulation. Critical analysis together with appropriate provision through a range of agencies has focused on the rights of children and young people to develop, explore and control their sexual destinies. Yet it has been the assumed relationship between physical development and social expectation which has had such a profound influence on the contradictory messages of sexual liberation and sexual protection. Within this broader context significant social policy and legal changes occurred throughout the 1980s and 1990s. They included the issue of 'Gillick competence', the purpose, role and scope of sex education in schools, the political dynamics and consequences of Section 28 and the Age of Consent debates. These developments and the media and political debates which raged around them are considered before moving to an examination of a children's rights approach to sex and sexuality.

The issues raised in the chapter on sexuality are closely aligned to the key themes examined in the chapter on schools and schooling. While the legislation governing education in Britain provides for children and young people to be tutored at home or in fee-paying residential schools, the majority attend compulsory day schools from the ages of 5 to 16. Late nineteenth century educational reforms were seen as progressive and enabling insofar as children, for the first time, received formal education as an integral part, if not right, of childhood. Traditional theories of education, while diverse, broadly accepted that the function of school was to prepare children and young people for 'life' and adulthood, ensuring the acquisition of 'appropriate' knowledge, skills, attitudes and values in a structured and disciplined environment. What was deemed *appropriate*, however, was determined primarily by the correspondence, in terms of curriculum relevance and 'appropriate' skills, between schooling and work. While this broad framework has prevailed, critical approaches have challenged the consensual representation of schooling, exposing the formal processes as regulatory and determining, derived in and reflective of broader structural inequalities within the political economy. The power relations inherent within a society, which excludes, marginalizes or denies children, become part of the operational context of education, in curriculum (formal and informal), organization, interpersonal relations and 'acceptable' behaviour. The development of educational policies is traced from the late nineteenth century through to current reforms. A key tension in the theory and practice of schooling is the relationship of the principle of 'education for all' with hierarchical provision based on selection and related directly to a society in which inequalities are all-pervasive. From the early commitment to universal schooling through to the postwar rhetoric of equal educational opportunity within the context of a rising meritocracy, the chapter shows that 'progressive' educational philosophy was developed and envisaged early in the twentieth century but has never been adopted universally. The reaffirmation of traditional principles and the attack on pluralist ideals concerning 'consensus' became hallmarks of the New Right agenda brought to fruition by successive Thatcher administrations. The full range of recent education reform is considered and critiqued in the context of a rights approach to children and schooling.

The UK incarcerates more children and young people than any other state within the European Union. In 1993, following the killing of James Bulger, plans were announced to extend incarceration to include children as young as 12 and, accordingly, the 1994 Criminal Justice and Public Order Act established the Secure Training Order. Newly-built secure units will house this new age group of 'serious' offenders. The youth justice chapter locates the locking-up of children and young people within the broader theoretical context of punishment, imprisonment and regulation. It focuses on the contradictions between *care* and *protection*, considering the control and punishment of young people in the context of the welfare–justice debate. It considers the politics and processes of *responsibility*, as the *protection of the child* is replaced by populist assumptions and responses concerning the *protection of the public*. Significant here are the implications of contemporary social and legal policy changes for children in trouble. As discussed earlier, the current trend in Britain towards a 'get tough' response to troublesome children flies in the face of successful developments in youth justice throughout the 1980s and it has major consequences and ramifications for the lives of children and young people.

Troublesome children have not only provided the bread and butter for a whole range of welfare and child-care professionals, they have also led to the pathologizing and medicalization of children's behaviours. Perhaps the most permissive and extensive power assumed by adults-as-professionals over children-as-problems is the discretion of classification. In defining and responding to children and young people as '*disturbed*' or '*disturbing*', in utilizing dubious methodologies in the pursuit of 'scientific' classification, adults use their professional powers to insist on the modification of behaviours assumed to be deviant. The chapter on mental health is centrally concerned with the theoretical 'knowledge' and professional discourses emanating from the academic disciplines of psychology and psychiatry. It is from within these discourses that the arbiters of 'normality' have emerged since the mid-nineteenth century. They have provided 'scientific' legitimation to state policies and practices of social regulation and health-care reform. Significant within these developments have been the determining contexts and social constructions of the mental health of children and young people. Consequently, the chapter considers the contemporary debates on the perceived deterioration in the mental health of children and young people, particularly its association with assumptions of increased violence and lawlessness. In this climate, however, the state's response to 'disturbed' or 'disturbing' children has not been consistent. State policy and professional practice has neglected safeguards for the protection of those so defined and this systematic denial of rights has enabled a wide range of institutional and personal abuse perpetrated by adult carers.

This is not an optimistic book. One unambiguous conclusion to be drawn from the wealth of material and argument on which it draws is that in British society many children are compelled to live a lie. The lie is that this is a society which values, cares for and protects them – a society populated by families and served by institutions in which they are safe and unthreatened. In deconstructing the adult myth that 'childhood' is in 'crisis' the concluding chapter revisits the relationship between the structural determinants of '*childhood*' and the experiential world of children. It questions the means through which adultism becomes institutionalized and mediated through social structures and their processes and policies. Important to this evaluation are the ways in which material power is complemented by persistent ideologies of subservience and subjugation to silence the voices and nullify the actions of young people. Nowhere has this silence been more apparent, more conspicuous, than in the debates of the 1990s. No other group of people could have been so systematically ignored, banished from the forums without a second thought. It is this sequence which elevates adultism, as an oppressive material and intellectual force, above ageism. The former is specific only to children and young people. Thus the argument for a critical theory of childhood is made not only as a response to and critique of the academic traditions and the 'back to basics' rhetoric of the New Right, but also as a rejection of the self-styled 'ethical socialists' previously mentioned.

Undoubtedly, there are significant social problems concerning children and young people which need to be considered in their complexity. The recent resurgence of well-worn, unsophisticated academic traditions coupled with political rhetoric often verging on bigotry, however, has resulted in an aggressive authoritarianism only compounding the alienation experienced by children and young people. It has been this depiction of a 'crisis' in 'childhood', threatening the very fabric of the social and moral order, so powerful, so pervasive, so punishing, that has masked the structural and material realities which oppress young people and institutionally deny them access to basic rights and civil liberties. Yet, despite the persistence and intensity of this political pressure, their denial has been resisted by young people and by those who work closely alongside them. In a climate in which essential services have been subjected to swingeing cuts in resources, there have been pockets of commitment from within the professions and voluntary organizations to the maintenance of sound, critical practice. Advocacy agencies, both regional and national, involving children and young people have used the more potentially progressive policy and legal reforms to challenge the powers vested in adulthood. Children and young people themselves have demonstrated their resilience and initiative in resisting the determining processes which seek to exclude them. A significant support to this resistance is the UN Convention on the Rights of the Child and the criticism levelled against the British Government by the UN Committee in not implementing its Articles. It is towards the tangible and realizable objectives contained within a rights perspective and politics that the work which follows is committed.

Young People, Power and Justice Research Group
Centre for Studies in Crime and Social Justice
Edge Hill University College
July 1996

Acknowledgements

The Young People, Power and Justice Research Group was founded in 1993 as one of five research groups at the Centre for Studies in Crime and Social Justice, Edge Hill University College. It brought together researchers active in teaching, social work, child protection, youth justice and higher education. Their common concern, following the killing of James Bulger and the subsequent trial of two young boys for his murder, was the unprecedented media, political and professional reaction towards children in general. 'Childhood', it was argued, was in a state of 'crisis'. The Group focused on the social construction of 'childhood', the formation of dominant ideologies and their impact on legislation, state policies and professional practices. It created a critical forum for the initiation and administration of research and in March 1994 held a one-day regional conference for people working with or campaigning alongside children and young people.

The 'Childhood' in 'Crisis'? conference was highly successful, combining plenary contributions with practice-based workshops. We are grateful to the conference participants for their part in developing the key themes and in giving their time, interest and commitment to the issues. They also provided clear evidence of the shared struggles and resistances which have evolved to challenge adultism within professional agencies and state institutions. Our thanks are also due to Andrew O'Hagan for his introductory plenary which contextualized the 'crisis' and to Jane Dalrymple and Rachel Cross of the non-statutory, children's rights and representation agency, Advocacy Services for Children. Their plenary on rights, responsibilities and resistances was a vital contribution. The conference provided the stimulus to develop further the key themes for research and publication. This book is one direct outcome of the conference, expanding and consolidating its principal themes.

We would like to thank Elaine Rawlinson, who participated in the group's early meetings. Ingrid Hall had a formative role in the group's work and direction and she contributed significantly to the conference organization and workshops. We also want to acknowledge the continual support of our colleagues at the Centre for Studies in Crime and Social Justice, particularly Kathryn Chadwick, Margaret Malloch and the forum for critical analysis and constructive debate offered by the Centre's Advanced Research Group. Barbara Houghton, the Centre Coordinator, provided the full range of administrative expertise and personal support required for organizing conferences, group meetings and subsequent publications, including word-processing this text. We are grateful for the patient encouragement and professional advice given by our colleagues at Taylor and Francis, particularly Comfort Jegede, who commissioned the book, Fiona Kinghorn, Sheena Sukumaran and Alison Chapman.

The chapters are primarily the responsibility of the authors. Our intention has been to use the collective discussions and research of the Group as the foundation for writing each chapter. Editing the chapters has focused on developing the main themes within an integrated and coherent framework established through our meetings. This is not an exercise in writing '*for*' or '*on behalf of*' children and young people. Like the continuing work of the Young People, Power and Justice Research Group, it represents a critical review and analysis of the contemporary mainstream debate which has sought to exclude and marginalize children and young people, their views, experiences and aspirations.

> Phil Scraton (on behalf on the Young People,
> Power and Justice Research Group)
> Merseyside
> July 1996

Chapter 1

'Childhood': An Introduction to Historical and Theoretical Analyses

Barry Goldson

The individual confronts society when he (sic) is still in the cradle. The baby's cry . . . becomes the individual's first contact with the surrounding world; it forges the link in the long chain that constitutes the social order.

(Rousseau, 1756)

What is Childhood?: Some Preliminary Thoughts

The dominant and prevailing western representation of childhood conceptualizes an idealized world of innocence and joy; a period of fantastic freedom, imagination and seamless opportunity. Children are thought to occupy the space provided by a 'walled garden' which protects them from 'the harshness of the world outside' (Holt, 1975:22). The adult–child relation is said to provide protection: serving the 'best interests of the child' and meeting 'children's needs'. The adult is guardian and is charged with responsibility for the child's welfare. Such popular understanding and cultural representation is underpinned by a particular form of what Shamgar-Handelman (1994:250) refers to as 'emotional, value-laden and moralistic rhetoric' which accommodates an 'unquestioning, complacent acceptance of whatever social, educational and political arrangements have arisen to cope with them [children]' (Scarre, 1989:x). This childhood 'reality' is questionable, demanding critical evaluation. Accordingly, concepts such as the 'good of the child', the 'best interests of the child' and 'children's needs' have been challenged (Rodham, 1976), as have idealistic representations of childhood as an unproblematic period of innocence, freedom, limited responsibility and minimal obligations (Postman, 1982; Winn, 1983). Moreover, the very nature and application of power which characterizes the child–adult relation and the uncritical acceptance of the protective imperative cannot be sustained.

Understanding the child–adult relation as an exclusively benign and consensual arrangement, guaranteeing and protecting the interests of the child is problematic. Shamgar-Handelman observes that, childhood is that period during which persons are subject to a set of rules and regulations unique to them, and one that does not apply to members of other social categories. Moreover, childhood is a period in a person's life during which he/she is neither expected nor allowed to fully participate in various domains of social life (1994:251).

This analysis moves the focus from notions of protection to concepts of exclusion, regulation and subordination whereby the 'walled garden' is reconstructed in a form within which childhood is experienced 'not as a garden but as a prison' (Holt, 1975:23), or what Gura (1994:102) describes as a 'virtual ghetto . . . a world cut off from the interests and activities of society at large'. This is not a world of freedom and opportunity but one of confinement and limitation in which children are 'wholly subservient and dependent', being seen as 'a mixture of expensive nuisance, slave and super-pet' (Holt, 1975:15). Further, this can be a world of isolation, sadness, exploitation, oppression, cruelty and abuse (Campbell, 1988; Hall and Lloyd, 1993; Miller, 1990).

To dichotomize and juxtapose these theoretical models of the child–adult relation reveals fundamentally different ways of seeing and understanding the very essence of contemporary childhood. Paradoxically, however, such models as far as they are developed here, are essentially similar in that they rest implicitly on a biologically determined or naturalistic construction of childhood. In this context *childhood* is represented as a fact of human life with biology determining children's dependency on adults to provide care. The social, political and economic dimensions of the adult–child power relation are absent from this analysis. While immaturity and dependence may be biological facts of life, however, James and Prout (1990:7) contend that 'the ways in which this immaturity is understood and made meaningful is a fact of culture. It is these "facts of culture" which may vary and which can be said to make of childhood a social institution.' In this sense childhood is not a static, objective and universal fact of human nature, but a social construction which is both culturally and historically determined.

The conceptualization of childhood as a social, cultural and historical construction is derived in the work of the French historian Philippe Ariès who claims that in 'medieval society the idea of childhood did not exist', as once the 'child' moved from the biological dependence of 'infancy' it 'belonged to adult society' (Ariès, 1962:125). Drawing on a range of medieval cultural evidence, including diaries and paintings, Ariès contends that children were indiscernible from adults as they dressed, behaved and conversed similarly, and were engaged in the same social activities and work. Effectively, they were miniature adults. According to Ariès' analysis the concept of childhood as a discrete life stage emerged in Europe between the fifteenth and eighteenth centuries as part of a process driven by two primary imperatives. First, there was an affective or 'codlling' dimension 'in which the child, on account of his (sic) sweetness, simplicity and drollery, became a source of amusement and relaxation for the adult' (Ariès, 1962:126). Second, there was an educational dimension inspired by 'churchmen or gentlemen of the robe . . . moralists and peda-gogues' (Ariès, 1962:128–30) and advanced initially by the Calvinist priorities. This secured control over children's innate 'depravity' and was developed through the influence of the Reformation, with its emphasis on discipline and knowledge of theology, humanities and sciences. It was consolidated during the period of European Enlightenment with the ascendancy of 'rationality'. Initially restricted to the domain of upper-class childhood, Ariès contends that the affective and educational dimensions eventually diffused across society and childhood became institutionalized.

The definitive work of Ariès has not been without critique. It has been argued that his thesis under-estimated the nature of childhood within changing household structures and family forms (Gelis, 1986; Stone, 1974); his evidence was loose and over-simplistic (Frost and Stein, 1989); his analysis placed insufficient emphasis on economic changes and the context of class (Thane, 1981); his account negated the historical constancy of the parent–child relation characterized by love and affection (Pollock, 1983); although responses to children have shifted through history, childhood was not discovered in the way that Ariès suggested but has always comprised a human universal (De Mause, 1976). It is not the intention here, however, to scrutinize and evaluate the detail of Ariès' work but to acknowledge the profound significance of his contribution in presenting childhood as a social construction which challenged populist and intellectual orthodoxy (see Morel, 1989; Niestroj, 1989). As Holt observes:

> Those who have recently begun to study the origins and history of childhood appear to have learned that childhood, motherhood, home, family, all of these institutions as we know them, are in impor-tant respects local and recent inventions, not some universal part of the human condition (1975:28).

James and Prout add:

> Childhood is understood as a social construction . . . Childhood, as distinct from biological immaturity, is neither a natural nor universal feature of human groups but appears as a specific structural and cultural component of many societies. Childhood is a variable of social analysis. It can never be entirely divorced from other variables such as class, gender or ethnicity. Comparative and cross-cultural analysis reveals a variety of childhoods rather than a single and universal phenomenon (1990:8).

Historical analysis, involving identification, mapping and a critical exami-nation of the processes within which childhood is constructed, 'discovered' (Scarre, 1989:7) or 'invented' (Suransky, 1982) has been central to contempor-ary debates. While this has been a complex task, fraught with difficulties

(Jordanova, 1989; Pollock, 1983:65–6), it has formed the foundations on which to build critical analysis and to challenge prevalent ideologies and academic orthodoxies in relation to understanding children's experiences of childhood.

Childhood in History: Social Construction and Reconstruction

The central contention here is that at any historical moment childhood will be constructed around a complex interplay of competing social, economic and political priorities. This is not intended to negate the primary significance of biological relations, but to shift the focus from notions of naturalistic determinism to an analysis of the conceptual relativity of childhood within history. The limitations imposed here confine the historical analysis to a review of the constructions and reconstructions of childhood during the last two centuries.

The consolidation of industrial capitalism in the first half of the nineteenth century comprised, in the words of Tobias (1967:255) a 'society in violent economic and social transition'. Indeed, the simultaneous processes of mushrooming urbanization and industrialization, massive population shift and internal migration, a developing political consciousness and militancy among sections of the working class, and the proliferation of abject poverty, destitution and homelessness, were material manifestations of a period of unprecedented social, economic and political change (see Engels, 1968; Hobsbawn, 1968; Jenkins, 1980). Within this climate of flux and uncertainty the prevalent bourgeois construction of childhood and its concomitant 'domestic ideal' (Hendrick 1990b) had little relevance (or application) to the material realities of the working-class child.

The early capitalist economy required cheap labour and, as Morris and McIsaac (1978:2) note, 'statesmen, administrators and employers alike all turned to the child: the child was a source of industrial wealth.' Child labour was traditional, universal and inescapable and in the first decades of the nineteenth century, children were widely employed in textiles, mining, agriculture, domestic service, docks and navigation (Hunt, 1981). For example, 80 per cent of workers in English cotton mills were children (Gillis, 1974). Wintersberger notes:

> The subsumption of childhood under capital in 19th-century England was described in all its brutality . . . reports of factory inspectors and children's employment commissioners as well as from public health reports, provide a realistic picture of the condition of working class children in the most advanced industrial country of its time . . . Children, sometimes not older than seven years of age, were working more than ten hours a day . . . they were exploited as cheap labour under the worst and most unhealthy conditions (1994:216).

As the century progressed, however, a developing humanitarianism and revulsion against the working conditions of the child combined to initiate reform movements opposing child exploitation. The 1833 Factories Act limited the conditions under which children could be employed (Pike, 1966; Pinchbeck and Hewitt, 1969). While the Act can be interpreted as humane and progressive in liberating urban children from the most barbaric forms of industrial bondage, it served also to compound their marginalization and impoverishment. Wintersberger (1994:213) notes that 'as their contributions to the (national and domestic) economy vanished, children seem to have disappeared as subjects and actors.' Further, the urban juvenile population rapidly exceeded the restricted employment opportunities bringing a serious escalation of child vagrancy and unemployment. Without employment opportunities, children were often abandoned and this swelled the poor population leaving unsupervised children adrift on the streets.

Indeed, the so-called 'advances' of industrialization and urbanization had serious consequences. Displacement of communities, structured unemployment and socio-political unrest resulted in marginalization and abandonment of many working-class children whose 'opportunities' were restricted to petty offending as the means of survival. Effectively, the 'factory child' was replaced by the 'delinquent child' (Hendrick, 1990b, 1994). Muncie notes:

> Whether or not the state of delinquency was in fact increasing is statistically unanswerable . . . but it was clear that it was contemporary conviction that the crime rate was rising and that juveniles should be protected both from themselves and from contamination by those already engaged in criminal 'capers' (1981:14).

The ideological construction of juvenile delinquency reflected the emergence and consolidation of moral anxieties and reactionary political concerns. Concepts of immorality, irreligion, corruption and contagion combined with constructs of dangerousness, sedition and political subversion and were frequently applied in analyses of crime in general, and juvenile crime in particular (Ignatieff, 1978; Pearson, 1975, 1983; Thompson, 1968). Moral panic and political reaction dovetailed into a developing bourgeois philanthropic tendency which mobilized charity crusades and inspired voluntary effort. The Society for Investigating the Causes of the Alarming Increase of Juvenile Delinquency in the Metropolis, which emerged from a voluntary initiative in 1815, served as a catalyst for a wave of similar effort and concern, galvanizing the 'child rescue movement'. Championed by Mary Carpenter and her philanthropic contemporaries, the 'movement' gathered momentum driven by their writings, public meetings and practical experiments and fuelled by the prevailing moral panic and political concern (Carpenter, 1851, 1853). Carpenter's efforts became institutionalized through the emergence of Reformatories and Industrial Schools, receiving legislative sanction in 1854 and 1857 respectively.

Reformatories and industrial schools were established and developed to stem the 'rising tide' of juvenile delinquency by providing institutional regimes geared primarily to the imposition of moral rectitude. The reformatories received children of the 'dangerous classes' aged 16 years and under and convicted of an offence punishable by imprisonment or penal servitude. The industrial schools received children of the 'perishing classes', those found begging or receiving alms, wandering and not having any home or visible means of subsistence. The emergence of these institutions was fundamental in the deconstruction of the childhood of labour, agrarian and industrial bondage and in the reconstruction of childhood informed by the imperatives of moral correction, regulation, protection, subservience and subordination. The reformatories and industrial schools were institutional responses to 'justice' and 'welfare needs', embodying the separation of 'depraved' from 'deprived' children and of the 'undeserving' from the 'deserving'. Moreover, they were institutional manifestations of a reconstructed childhood, captured in the words of Hill when, in 1855, he wrote that the delinquent

> is a little stunted man already – he knows much and a great deal too much of what is called life – he can take care of his own immediate interests. He is self-reliant, he has so long directed or mis-directed his own actions and has so little trust in those about him, that he submits to no control and asks for no protection. He has consequently much to unlearn – he has to be turned again into a child (in Hendrick, 1990b:43).

As Hendrick observes, 'here was a critical turning point in the history of age relations . . . for under construction was a carefully defined "nature", one that posed a return to an earlier mythical condition of childhood' (1990b:43). The socio-economic transition which substituted the 'factory child' by the 'delinquent child' created a residuum, a surplus population of children for whom society had no legitimate space. 'Child-saving' filled this vacuum and prioritized 'resocialization'. This was a process that necessitated 'unlearning', a process involving the restoration of what Carpenter called 'the true position of childhood . . . a child is to be treated as a child' (quoted in Manton, 1976:109).

If the reformatories and industrial schools emerged as responses to delinquency and destitution it was education that consolidated the processes of resocialization and moral correction. Schooling initially developed as the *ad hoc* provision for middle-class children, increasingly educated to secondary level. Opportunities for working-class children, however, were restricted to reformatories, charity schools, Sunday schools, ragged schools or poor law district schools (Emsley, 1987:57). It was not until 1870 that the state took responsibility for the schooling of all 'able-bodied' children. The 1870 Education Act introduced the state into child-rearing practices, socialization and the conceptualization of a 'national childhood'. Education for all, and a commitment to the 'schooled child', became important factors in the shaping and structuring of a new childhood. Children, no longer active workers and industrial participants, were required to become passive pupils and learning subordinates (Rose, 1991). Hendrick notes:

> There is no doubt that in the last quarter of the nineteenth century the school played a pivotal role in the construction of a new kind of childhood . . . the classroom and the ideological apparatus of education were crucial because they demanded – indeed could not do without – a truly national childhood . . . this construction directly involved all children . . . and was intended to be inescapable (1990b:46).

At the end of the nineteenth century Britain was further absorbed in fundamental socio-economic change within which the role of the state was again being redefined and renegotiated. New industrial and labour relations, the widening of markets and the intensification of foreign competition, the demands of the Empire, the continued development of organized labour and the maturing politicization of the working class were the material complexities to which the state had to respond. Despite economic expansionism, however, disadvantage and poverty endured alongside improved standards of living. These were the dynamics and tensions that characterized the central objective of government: maintaining economic and social stability at home while securing administrative domination of the colonies. Britain was negotiating its place within an emerging world economic, social and political order and it was a time of great uncertainty which inevitably affected children as 'philanthropy took second place to unadulterated imperialism (and children) were thought of as "Bricks for Empire Building"' (Bean and Melville, 1989:78).

The ascendancy of Social Darwinism and the eugenics movement focused attention on the importance of creating and sustaining the conditions within which children could develop healthily for the 'good of the nation'. The gaze turned to physicality and the body, and the school became an observational locus both for monitoring and inspecting the child's body and in arranging for its treatment (see Armstrong, 1983; Rose, 1985). Hendrick (1990b:47) notes that the school provided opportunities 'to doctors who, in common with sociologists, psychologists, educationalists and philanthropic reformers, used the classroom as a laboratory in which to produce "scientific" surveys of the pupils.' While attention was previously concerned with specific groups of children, primarily the neglected and the delinquent, the school widened the net to include the entire school age population.

Within this context child psychology and the child-study movement emerged and developed, forming the basis of a new authoritative scientism. Inextricably linked to the new scientism, grounded in psychology, was a broader developing interest in child welfare. The 1906 Education (Provision of Meals) Act empowered local authorities to feed children at school and the following year the Education (Provisions) Act placed a duty on local authorities to examine medically all children attending elementary school. The 1907 Notification of Births Act provided for the compulsory registration of children and the introduction of health visitors. Also in 1907 the Probation of Offenders Act reformed and humanized criminal law in relation to children and the 1908 Children Act consolidated previously fragmented law, offering greater protection from cruelty and abuse to children. In 1909 the Royal Commission on the Poor Law condemned the use of workhouses for children and in 1913 a Poor Law Institutions Order imposed far-reaching limitations on workhouses in respect of children. The implementation of these, and other measures, provided both for the emergence of state welfare bureaucracies and the developing universal concept of a *national childhood* ostensibly derived in notions of vulnerability and the need for protection.

The convergence of the new scientism, rooted in psychology and state-led provision and framed within welfare legislation, not only shaped the definition of the 'national child' but manifested a consciously designed and focused pursuit of national interest, demanding efficiency, public health, education, order, conformity and protection. Children were regarded as a source of raw material, a national asset which required some nurturing and investment. As Hendrick (1994:4) perceptively comments:

> The understanding and serving of children did not develop from unblemished altruistic motives. In an age of fierce imperial, political, military and economic national rivalries, in addition to domestic anxieties regarding class politics, urban hygiene, and social stability, children were indeed promises of wealth, power and opportunities.

It is within this context of domestic and international uncertainty that a construction of national childhood informed by a developing professional discourse, with its primary emphasis on the healthy body, emerged in the years leading up to the First World War.

The developing constructions of childhood throughout the 1920s and 1930s were not consistent. Economic depression and widespread unemployment were inevitably accompanied by government financial retrenchment, inherent poverty, poor housing and ill-health. The earlier emphasis on the health and welfare of the 'national child', underpinned by the priorities associated with military and industrial efficiency at home and abroad, was diluted. Macnicol notes, 'It is hardly surprising that in the inter-war years, when this militaristic fervour had waned and a vast army of unemployed provided a pool of surplus labour, there was less immediate concern over the health of future generations' (1980:44). Within government there was inevitable resistance to a programme of open-ended investment and welfare spending at a time of economic crisis. As Macnicol states, attempts to establish the principle of minimum standards were obstructed:

the evidence of poverty and malnutrition in large families slowly grew . . . this evidence was repeatedly presented to the government . . . yet the government steadfastly denied that there was any pressing need to raise the economic status of mothers and children . . . the government was clearly determined not to announce a minimum needs level in cash terms, for to do so would open the way to demands that a large section of the working class . . . should have their incomes brought up to such a level. This was something to be resisted at all costs (1980:66–7).

Although economic retrenchment and calculated financial expediency comprised an imposing context, it did not, of itself, result in the abandonment of the constructions of childhood that were developing within professional discourse and the professional institutionalization and colonization of childhood throughout the inter-war period. Psychology, psychiatry, education, health and welfare imperatives combined to form the steadily developing, if contested, terrain of professional knowledge and discourse concerning children and childhood. Significantly, such developments brought a re-orientation of emphasis as professional interest expanded its focus from an exclusive concern with medical and material welfare to include more overtly psychological and psychiatric paradigms. The *body* was now accompanied by the *mind* as three cornerstone principles were established: the mind of the child; the child and the family; child management (Cooter, 1992; Rose, 1985).

Despite retrenchment, economic crisis and depression Stevenson and Cook argue that children's health was generally improved by diet, better housing and sanitation:

In spite of setbacks in the depressed areas, the decade after 1929 saw a continuation of the progress which had been made in public health since the First World War. By 1939 Britain was a healthier nation . . . than it had been ten years earlier, in spite of many problems which still required attention (1994:27–8).

Also, child health continued to be monitored and routinely inspected by the School Medical Service (Rose, 1991:158–60). It was the emergence and application of psychological and psychiatric frameworks, however, and the professional popularization of psychoanalysis which contributed significantly to constructions of childhood during the inter-war period. As Hendrick (1990b, 1994), Riley (1983), and Rose (1985, 1990) note, the work of Burt, Isaacs, Klein, Bowlby and Freud, although not consensual, nonetheless had a profound collective impact as 'new' knowledges bolstered professional power and authority. The mind of the child became the subject of inquiry and central to this development was the child guidance movement.

The central, operational brief of the Child Guidance Council was the responsibility to 'treat' 'maladjusted', 'difficult', and 'delinquent' children. This represented an institutional expression of a growing concern with national mental health and the psychiatric delineation of childhood's 'specific repertoire of disorders'. The Child Guidance Clinic had both preventive and treatment objectives in identifying 'maladjustment' and assisting families in developing the conditions within which it could be avoided and 'cured'. Moreover, it evidenced the influence of psychology and the shift from *body* to include *mind*, and represented a more subtle and calculated form of state investment. As Urwin and Sharland (1992:191) note, 'The neglected toddler in everyone's way is the material which becomes the disgruntled agitator, while the happy contented child is the pillar of the state.'

The guidance clinics, alongside other professional developments, gave early expression both to the 'problem child' and to the 'problem family' or 'bad family' in need of rehabilitation and state intervention. The discovery of what Hendrick (1990b) calls the 'psychological child' and the professional reorientation which embraced both body and mind comprises a significant period in terms of the relation between the child, the family and the state. The boundaries which had previously enveloped the essentially private domain of the family were under negotiation as state agencies sought to define and claim interventionist space.

The sense of optimism within Britain, and the promise of a renewed social order which prevailed in 1945, was galvanized within the period of post-war reconstruction and provided the foundations on which planning for democratic families, 'problem families' and the comprehensive reorganization of welfare services would develop. Childhood was central to this period of reconstruction. Informed largely by cross-class notions of the child as war victim (evacuation; the blitz; trauma; slums and decay; destruction and separation) public and political priorities were given to the creation of a social democracy within which the child and the family would be guaranteed security. The welfare state derived in Beveridge, together with Macmillan's 1950s paternalistic, 'never had it so good' oratory underpinned a unique period of state interventionism and centralized management of the economy. The social contract and high levels of employment heralded the arrival of the 'affluent worker' (Goldthorpe, Lockwood, Bechofer and Platt, 1969). Similarly, the demands of new forms of production and promise of upward, social mobility witnessed the emergence of the nuclear family (Willmott and Young, 1986). A new, and apparently consensually based, welfare capitalism promised a comprehensive range of health, education, housing, social security and personal social services which would sustain a healthy childhood within the healthy family (Frost and Stein, 1989; Gough, 1979; Marsh, 1980; Marshall, 1965).

The commitment to the child as an investment was pre-eminent in post-war politics, and the perceived value of children had two specific inflexions. First, as Hendrick notes:

> In the case of the family, the importance of the child was as a properly functioning member of a properly functioning group – in other words, the child was important for itself in the present; its healthy emotional and physical development was evidence of the harmonious domestic environment (1994:285).

Here the child represented a barometer of the post-war national health. Second, the child was important as an investment for the purpose of securing the nation's future. Children were personified as a key form of national insurance, a developing source of labour, professional activity and expertise. The family, particularly the emerging nuclear or conjugal unit, was seen as the primary organizational institution to nurture and socialize the child. And women were to return to the home as mothers, carers and socializers.

The unequivocal perception of the importance of the family was, of course, informed by pre-war and war-time experiences. Heywood (1959:134) argues that the relative success with which the family endured the formidable challenges of the war was evidence of the 'extraordinary strength, tenacity and satisfaction found in the family group'. This observation combined with inter-war psychoanalytic psychology and child-guidance philosophy which proclaimed that the family, particularly the parent (mother) – child relationship, was invaluable to healthy childhood (Bowlby, 1953, 1988). Such a combination had substantial influence not only in defining a primary caring role for women as mothers and wives, but also in constructing an image of children as vulnerable, requiring protection, dependent, innocent, malleable, subordinate and in need of adult guidance, direction and socialization.

The emphasis on the healthy family, however, almost by definition provided a construction of its converse, the 'unhealthy', 'dysfunctional', 'problem', 'bad' or 'dangerous' family. This legitimized state intervention into a hitherto private world. The 1948 Children Act, and the establishment of the Children's Service, created new and organizationally autonomous children's departments, thus severing the administrative heritage of the Poor Law. The new departments employed children's officers who adopted a social casework model serving to justify formal state intervention into the privacy of family life. The Act placed a clear responsibility on local authorities to provide for children in public care but it also required children's departments to maintain and nurture the child's links with their natural family and, wherever possible, return the child to that family. Similarly, the Curtis Committee Report, which led directly to the 1948 Act, concluded that the institutional care of children was damaging and should be replaced by 'the free conditions of ordinary family life' provided, if necessary, by foster care (see Frost and Stein, 1989:33–4; Parton, 1985). These postwar welfare developments, therefore, not only constructed a clearer concept of the 'public child' but also reaffirmed the ideology of the functional family and the domestic ideal: state departments were given the responsibility for reparatory interventions aimed to 'rehabilitate' and 'reconstitute' natural families or to identify substitute families. While welfare departments emerged as 'sensitive to the emotional needs of children' (Pinchbeck and Hewitt, 1973:647) they also served to construct an ideology of national childhood in which the family was seen as imperative, with children being the property of their parents.

Subsequent developments within the broader context of welfare state provision confirmed the structural relation between the child, the family and the state. This is not to suggest, however, that childhood was firmly established and static. Although contemporary professional discourse and knowledge (encompassing law, medicine, psychiatry, psychology, education, social work) reflects an ideology of childhood based on innately and structurally vulnerable minors requiring protection, definitions of childhood are consistently negotiated and revised. The child as *victim* (the 'battered baby' of the 1960s; the 'abused child' of the 1970s; the 'sexually abused child' of the 1980s and 1990s), in the words of Hendrick (1994:286), has taken its place 'in the gallery of social constructions which paradoxically reveal the monumental indifference of adults to this form of child persecution throughout the greater part of the last century'. Conversely, the child as *threat* has been ever-present in different guises, recently re-emerging within the lexicon of such constructions: the child of 'yob culture' in need of resocialization via values of 'decency' and 'discipline' promised by a return to 'basics' (Goldson, 1994 and this volume). Central here has been the ascendancy and domination of the economics of Hayek and Friedman and its political institutionalization within the social policy of the New Right. The commitment to the dogma of the free market coupled with a fundamental hostility and malevolence to publicly funded welfare services and an entrenched belief in *laissez-faire* imperatives and individual responsibility were at the base of economic libertarianism. *Competitive individualism* became a euphemism for the economics of greed, deepening and widening structural divisions and resurrecting the imagery of the undeserving poor. Systematically entire communities and identifiable groups have been pathologized. Taken together, these political, economic and social developments have had serious consequences for the experiences of children and constructions of childhood.

Theorizing History: Childhood and Social Control

While brief and schematic, this historical contextualization demonstrates the critique of biological determinist theories of childhood and the challenge of social constructionist theories which have identified childhood within its social, political, economic and cultural contexts. The above historical overview is concerned with British childhood and its changes over the past two hundred years. Hendrick accounts for each new construction of childhood during this period in chronological order:

the factory child, the delinquent child, the schooled child, the psycho-medical child, and the welfare child of the era just prior to the first world war. Between 1914 and the late 1950s further developments produced what might more accurately be described as two 'reconstructions', since they depended so much on their nineteenth century heritage, namely the child of psychological jurisdiction – meaning child guidance clinics, psychoanalysis, educational psychology, and Bowlbyism; and, secondly, the family child (which included the 'public' child, usually children in care) (1990b:36–7).

What the earlier historical overview reveals, however, are the dialectic and dynamic contradictions which have shaped childhood: the ideological tensions and imperatives of care and welfare, control and justice, family responsibility and socialization, and work and labour. This historical process, and its social, economic and political priorities over two centuries, has shaped a more coherent concept of childhood located within the family as the principal institutional influence and as the prime site for socialization. It has determined the nature of the relationship between the child, the family and the state, and it has created the essential rhetorical foundations of a *national* childhood for *all* children. The role of the state is mediated through a range of what Foucault (1977) identifies as 'disciplinary networks', not exclusively punitive or corrective through legal control and regulation (reformatories and industrial schools for example), but also through bureaucracies whose purpose is to manage and tutor children by identifying and promoting their 'best interests'. Medicine, psychology, psychiatry, education, law, social work, for example, provide a regulatory network – what Donzelot (1980) refers to as the 'tutelary complex' – which blurs the boundaries between 'care' and 'control'.

Jordanova (1989:3) draws attention to two popular misconceptions in the interpretation of historical analysis whereby either 'the past is often idealized and the present depicted as a decline', or, conversely, 'the past becomes barbaric and exploitative [and] the present enlightened.' Each perspective is frequently applied to the history of childhood in popular discourse. The former is often found in analyses of juvenile crime which confidently proclaim that children are getting worse and are beyond control, that they display no respect — unlike the idealized good old days. Equally, the second perspective in which society enjoys a consistent process of improvement, humanization and benign incrementalism often prevails in generic histories of childhood. Children in western Europe are no longer working in the dungeons of the earth mining coal with their bare hands, they are literate and numerate, relatively well nourished, in good health and enjoy, in most cases, protection and security. Inevitably each of these models, each of these ways of seeing contains some truth and legitimacy, but both are simplistic, crude, reductionist and atheoretical representations of history. It is necessary to theorize childhood and to examine critically the constructions and reconstructions of childhood within the broader context of social, economic and political order and the imperatives of social control. The critical theoretical project facilitates 'decoding, demystification [and] unmasking' necessary to examine the 'deeper reality behind surface appearance' (Cohen, 1983:107). By looking beyond what Wright (1979:11) refers to as the 'world at the level of appearances' and developing a macro-theoretical analysis, the social, economic and political dynamics that have combined to shape and construct childhood are considered as central.

The conventional populist view of historical constructions of childhood and institutional developments within child-care is located within an idealized conceptualization of history which represents the historical process as a record of consistent progress. Reformism is characterized as an entirely benevolent expression of philanthropy, altruism and social progress, and institutional developments are interpreted as manifestations of the victory of humanitari-anism over barbarity, of scientific knowledge over prejudice and irrationality. Histories of childhood exude this *progress model* and, as Cohen observes:

> The source material . . . can be found in all the official commissions, enquiries and reports . . . the journals, textbooks, work-shops and conferences which are ground out by the control system (power) and the academic establishment (knowledge) to which it is symbiotically linked (1985:90).

The progress model has particularly strong practical and intellectual roots in the reforming zeal of the nineteenth century and the philanthropic enterprise of early reformers such as Mary Carpenter (1851, 1853). Indeed, as Cohen (1983:105) remarks, 'its believers are the genuine heirs of the nineteenth century reform tradition.'

The abstract reform vision which is located uncritically at the heart of the progress model of childhood history is questionable. Good intentions, driven by enlightened benevolence, must be taken seriously but an analysis of their social origins, the economic and political interests behind them, their internal paradoxes and the nature of their appeal is essential. Indeed, such a critique demonstrates that constructions and reconstructions of childhood, and the institutional forms within which children are ordered and socialized, are sub-stantially more complex than concepts such as 'reform', 'progress', 'doing good', 'best interests', 'benevolence', 'philanthropy', 'enlightenment' and 'humanitarianism' might in themselves imply. As Qvortrup observes:

> As childhood as a social construction changes, so also does the nature and the patterns of control over it . . . children who in every society are by definition excluded from the power game, control childhood the least . . . There is no doubt that childhood is to a large extent dependency, but the dependency may take several forms – exactly depending on the kind of struggle between other adult interests (1994:14).

Rothman (1987, 1980) argues that historical process is driven by the continual tension and interplay between *conscience* (the well-intentioned plans of reformers) and *convenience* (the obdurate nature of social reality comprising both macro-level and micro-level imperatives, interests and priorities). Further, Rothman accounts for the development and universality of social institutions by appealing to the concept of 'segregation for socialization', whereby discipline, order, regulation and control are secured within both justice and welfare orientated institutions. By applying Rothman's theoretical constructs to childhood, therefore, the development of schooling and the concept of education for all, for example, can be seen as an expression of conscience mediated according to the prevailing levels of convenience, and within the context of its socializing value.

In placing the relations of production at the centre of their analysis, Marxist writers emphasize the significance of contemporary class relations and their inherent contradictions to an understanding and interpretation of all aspects of social life within advanced capitalist political–economies. Within this theoretical model ideology is important not in itself, but because it enables the characterization of a coercive system as fair and humane. Here, historical constructions and reconstructions of childhood are contextualized within the demands of capital, and welfare ideology comprises a facade to present an acceptable face of the exercise of otherwise unacceptable power, domination and naked class interests. Cohen (1983:106) proposes that, 'Ideology is important only insofar as it succeeds at passing off as fair, natural, acceptable or even just, a system which is basically coercive.'

Similarly, Rusche and Kirchheimer (1938) have argued that welfare rhetoric disguises coercive developments which are determined by the demands of changing socio-economic structures. For them a primary purpose of reform was the need for more sophisticated methods of domination and discipline to serve the needs of developing industrial capitalism. As Cohen states:

> The control system continued to replicate and perpetuate the forms needed to serve its original purpose: ensuring the survival of the capitalist social order. The only real changes are those required by the evolving exigencies of capitalism: changes in the mode of production, fiscal crises, phases of unemployment, the requirements of capital. The theory of change is unambiguously materialist: knowledge, theory and ideology are generated as instruments to serve ruling class interests (1983:107).

Materialist theories of social change and social control resonate throughout historical analyses of childhood. Humanizing the working conditions of children, developments in schooling and education, improved health services and emphasis on both body and mind, welfare developments and public care and the formalized relation of the family and the state were each fundamental to the demands of capital and regulation of class relations.

Foucault (1977) shifts the focus both from abstract concepts of reform and progress and from the more materially determined accounts of historical process, social change and social control by analysing the compelling role of power in human motivation and human relations. For Foucault progress and humanism, good intentions, professional knowledge and reform rhetoric are neither in the idealist sense the producers of change, nor in the materialist sense the mere product of changes in the political economy. They are inevitably and inextricably linked to a 'power–knowledge spiral':

> We should not be content to say that power has a need for such-and-such a discovery, such-and-such a form of knowledge, but we should add that the exercise of power itself creates and causes to emerge new objects of knowledge and accumulates new bodies of information (Foucault in Gordon 1980:51).

Foucault's theoretical contentions focus on the notion of relentless 'discipline', the concept of power as ubiquitous and intrinsic to all human social relations and he emphasizes the mutual interdependence and inextricable interrelationship of power and knowledge. Power produces knowledge, but 'they imply one another', a site where power is exercised is also a place at which knowledge is produced. As Foucault states, 'there is no power relation without the correlative constitution of a field of knowledge that does not presuppose and constitute at the same time power relations' (1977:27). In applying such contentions to the historical processes within which childhood has been constructed and reconstructed, the synthesis of power and knowledge within professional discourse and the consequent development of what Foucault calls 'regimes of truth' or 'disciplinary networks' are of central importance. The professionalization of childhood and the emergence and development of discrete specialisms – each with its own corpus of knowledge and power – demands, maintains and reproduces a process whereby 'technicians' (doctors, psychiatrists, psychologists, teachers, social workers) have been able to penetrate and regulate the social world of the child. As Bardy observes:

> the voice of the professional has been raised, reflecting a wide spectrum of diversified specialization. Every major reform concerning children has been implemented through new, special groups of experts . . . Every profession dealing with children has its own specialised mandate, constructed in a given institution . . . Thus there is not only a network of adults but also a network of institutions devoted to childhood. A major part of childhood is compartmentalised in the institutions run by professional rationale . . . The social relations between minors and majors are, in everyday practice, embedded in professional (activity which serves to) 'convert' children into adults (1994:306).

In positioning the analysis of the historical constructions and reconstructions of childhood within a wider theoretical context the 'deeper reality behind surface appearance' (Cohen, 1983:107) is emphasized. While it is not the intention here to arbitrate between competing theoretical analyses of social change and control (epistemology, sociology of knowledge and materialist versus idealist versions of history) it is essential to acknowledge the tensions, the contested dynamics and the contradictions in and between different historical analyses of childhood. Different and competing theoretical perspectives can be outlined, albeit schematically, and contrasted. More difficult, however, is to extrapolate key principles from within and between these theoretical perspectives without falling into what Cohen (1985:112) refers to as 'the intellectual slush of "integration" in which all theories, ideas or philosophies imperceptibly merge with each other.'

With Cohen's cautionary message in mind, it is possible to identify elements of competing theoretical perspectives which, combined, can enhance the analysis of the social and historical construction of childhood. First, the *mind* has accompanied, if not replaced, the *body* as the primary site of intervention through private and public institutional forms of socialization. Second, the transitions and metamorphoses through which childhood has passed constitute more than the expression of humanitarian progress. Third, any notion of an abstract reform vision driving the processes of social change and social control is meaningless unless it is structurally located within the context of its historical antecedents, political interests, economic imperatives, cultural determinants, internal contradictions and practical applications. Fourth, welfare provision for children has emerged as part of a widening network of professional activity and aggrandizement within a centralized state apparatus to secure socialization, order and regulation. Fifth, institutions specifically for children have been developed and the inconsistencies and contradictions between rhetoric, regimes and reality can only be understood with reference to broader theoretical constructs. Sixth, each institutional form has developed its own body of 'expert' knowledge, adult knowledge, and the 'technicians', in expressing their professional authority and professional discretion, have established power both within the institutions and over their occupants. Finally, the control system has expanded and deepened relentlessly, securing a firm foothold within the private as well as the public domain.

Theoretical Specificity: The Structural Location of Childhood

Children and Adults: Rights, Power and Participation

The structural relation between children and adults is characterized by the institutional dependence of the former on the latter. This dominant organizational form permeates contemporary western society and is believed to be an essential social arrangement intrinsic to the natural order. The relation of dependence is thus naturalized and is invariably presented as entirely benign, with adults serving children's interest and meeting their needs. Adults are givers and providers, children are receivers and consumers; adults are protectors, children are protected; adults are thought to be mature, rational and strong, children are perceived as immature, irrational and vulnerable. Children grow into the world, steadily and incrementally they are integrated into society: childhood is a moratorium, a preparatory phase. James and Prout note:

> This dominant developmental approach to childhood . . . is a self-sustaining model whose features can be crudely delineated as follows: rationality is the universal mark of adulthood with childhood representing the period of apprenticeship for its development. Childhood is therefore . . . a pre-social period of difference, a biologically determined stage on the path to full human status, i.e., adulthood . . . It is essentially an evolutionary mode: the child developing into an adult represents a progression from simplicity to complexity of thought, from irrational to rational behaviour . . . acquisition of cognitive skill, into the social world of adults (1990:10–11).

The biological relation that exists between child and adult, together with its concomitant dependence, is rarely disputed although the exact nature and length of such a relation is both culturally and historically variable. Thus, to apply this construction universally, uncritically and unconditionally in all of its institutional forms is problematic in that it implies that children are not members – at least, not full members – of society. Indeed, children are reduced to the status of potential citizens: 'human becomings' as distinct from 'human beings' (Qvortrup, 1994:4).

This form of dependency-grounded, child–adult relation is consistent with Simone de Beauvoir's argument concerning the subject–object relationship as the basis of women's experience of 'otherness': 'She [woman] is defined and differentiated with reference to man, not he with reference to her . . . He is the Subject, He is the Absolute . . . She is the Other' (De Beauvoir, in Scraton, 1990:12) De Beauvoir's critical commentary on gender relations within patriarchy similarly can be applied to an analysis of the adult–child relation. Here the polarization of status is characterized by adults as subjects and children as objects, a state of 'otherness' within the over-arching context of adult hegemony. Such critical analysis problematizes the nature of the adult–child relation and raises fundamental questions concerning differential rights, power and participation within the determining context of generation. As Qvortrup (1994) contends, it challenges the principle of ontology and age, shaking the ideological foundation which legitimizes adults' natural right to exert power over children. Similarly, Bok notes:

As long as questions are not asked – as when power is thought divinely granted or ordained by nature – the right to coerce and manipulate is taken for granted. Only when this right is challenged does the need for justification arise. It becomes necessary to ask: when can authority be justly exercised over a child for instance (in Qvortrup 1994:3).

The moral or philosophical justification for the institutionalized exercise of adult power over children, in both the private and public domains, rests on three main requirements. First, a conception of the 'natural', as enduring, historically consistent and universal in the construction of the adult–child relation. Second, a cultural and consensual acceptance that the actor-status of adults is qualitatively more important than that of children. Third, unequivocal evidence that adults consistently exercise their power and authority and at all times behave in the best interests of children. However, the historical analysis of childhood shows that such requirements patently do not apply and are not met. Accordingly Qvortrup notes:

to the extent that adults and children are treated differently, dispose of different rights, are given different obligations, etc., the reason must be found somewhere else than in the ontological argument. The relationship between adults and children is therefore most likely not regulated philosophically, but by power and interest . . . children have no claim on equal treatment because they are not old enough (1991:4).

Indeed, age is a fundamental determinant in the distribution of rights, power and participation and children by virtue of their junior years and their institutional dependence on adults have limitations imposed upon their citizenship. The exact nature of the adult–child relation, as noted above, is historically constructed, but the principle of the object–subject dichotomy and the structural and institutional objectification and otherness of children endures.

Childhood as a Structural Division: Exclusion and Marginalization

The social, political and economic positioning of children in advanced capitalist economies is characterized by exclusion and marginalization. The adult–child relation does not simply confer protection *within* society. Children, it is claimed, must be protected *outside* society, and be shielded from the 'onerous responsibilities' of work, participation and influence. They are excluded from adult society and their marginalization is confirmed and guaranteed by legal obligation and the rule of law. As Bardy observes:

They are placed in 'waiting rooms', such institutions as schools, to become adults under the guidance and supervision of adults. As a consequence of this social exclusion, the dependency of minors on adults has become deeper and longer; consider, for example, the economic dependence because of the education required by society (1994:301).

Children are the only social group within the welfare state whose maintenance and care is primarily a private issue. They constitute in every sense a minority status and their structural exclusion and institutionalized marginalization renders them a 'muted group' (Hardman quoted in James and Prout, 1990:7). Thus childhood is a structural concept, a determining context (see Scraton and Chadwick, 1991), which may be analysed and understood alongside other structural forms and divisions within society, including class, 'race', gender, sexuality and disability. Further, as discrete structural division, childhood is particularly disadvantaged as children are denied access to the conventional sources of power, influence and authority in a liberal democracy. The relation of dependence which harnesses childhood to adulthood inevitably confirms its subservience and subordination. Childhood relies on adulthood, not only interpersonally, but also institutionally. Its structural exclusion and disenfranchisement is particularly marked here and is compounded by shifts in demographic patterns and social arrangements. As Qvortrup concludes:

> At one broad societal level children seem to be in the defensive to the extent that their share of the population in industrial countries for decades has been diminishing. This . . . reduces their likelihood to make claims on social resources with any strength; as a tendency – at least in numerical terms – children have fewer and fewer allies. A rapidly diminishing part of adults live together with children, and therefore the number of the electorate which has nothing at stake as far as children are concerned, is growing (1994:18).

Intra-Structural Divisions: The Concept of Childhoods

While it is necessary to theorize childhood as a discrete structural division and claim for it a legitimate space within the context of more established forms of sociological and structural analysis, it is equally important to embrace the fundamental issue that not all children experience childhood in the same way. The primary emphasis here is not with the *individual* child – although this has a value of its own – but with the *structural conditions* within which each childhood is determined: the relations of class, 'race', gender and sexuality. In other words, it is necessary to recognize intra-structural divisions and relations within the context of inter-structural analysis. Consequently, there is a range of childhoods: working-class, middle-class, black, white, male, female, homosexual, heterosexual, 'able bodied' and 'disabled', together with the complex permutations between and within these broader structural categories. Emphasis is placed here on what is common within childhood over what is unique to specific childhoods although it is essential to foreground the complexity of the plurality of childhoods in any focused institutional analysis (see, for example, Brown, 1990; Chisholm, 1990; Engelbert, 1994; Engler, 1990; Jones and Wallace, 1990; Krüger, 1990; Shamgar-Handelman, 1994, each of whom emphasizes the complex structuring and dynamics of internal differentiation and intra-structural division).

Processes of State Socialization: Time, Space and Specialist Institutions

Having discussed the constructs of power and authority underpinning the adult–child relation and established childhood as a structural form, it is important to consider the relations of childhood and the state. The welfare state has created public space for children comprising specialist institutions, some of which (i.e. schools) they are *required* by law to attend – or at least adults with parental responsibility are required by law to ensure that they attend – and others which are *available* to them. It is assumed that such institutions serve children's interests – caring, developmental, educational – in providing safe and secure time and space. This perspective dominates the progress model of historical development and social change. Specialist institutions, however, also provide for the exercise and influence of state power over children as Shamgar-Handelman observes when considering schooling:

> Within the framework of these educational institutions, persons spend much of their childhood period. In these educational frameworks, the children 'belong' to the state–society, and it is the state-supervised educational system that serves as a tool for the transmission of state-selected information, as well as values and norms (1994:262).

Thus schools socialize children towards legitimate adulthood; the state assumes *loco parentis*, transmits its message (the national curriculum) to a captive audience, and prepares its charges for social responsibility and work experience in society (Brown, 1987; Coles, 1995; Dale, 1985). Indeed, as Qvortrup (1994:10) notes, 'if schools were to be seen as society's courtesy towards children, we would be at pains to explain why schooling is obligatory.'

This form of analysis not only presents a critical challenge to dominant conceptions of specialist welfare institutions, it also raises questions concerning the time and space allocated to children within contemporary society. Ennew (1994) contends that children are 'ghettoized' and 'spatially outlawed' from modern society, and Kovarik (1994) develops the intriguing concepts of *stage* and *script* in his analysis of the spatial and temporal dimensions of childhood. The 'stage' refers to the design and structure of location while the 'script' is the agenda which determines the activity within a given stage. Such conceptions are consistent with the exclusion and marginalization of children from core societal activity, and their structural location on child-specific islands which serve to prepare the child/human *becoming* for the moment where he or she develops into the adult/human *being*.

The operational 'script' of the specialist institutions which engage children is set and managed invariably by welfare professionals and pedagogues whose discourse offers rhetorical constructions of their activity. Indeed, as noted, official representations of such institutions place their emphasis on benign child-centred priorities and employ an evocative and persuasive professional language to legitimize their forms of activity and intervention. It is the anaesthetizing function of professional language, within what is essentially a control system for children, which is of interest here, language employed, in the words of Orwell (1954:245), 'not so much to express meanings as to destroy them'. This is what Garland and Young (1983:18), in analysing criminal justice systems, have referred to as the political power of language to forge a distinction between the 'public realm of representation, significations and symbolic practices and the operational realm of sanctions, institutions and practices'. Similarly, Edelman (1977:16–20) refers to 'mythic cognitive structures' which manage through 'metaphor, metonymy and syntax to convey rhetorical evocations very far from their actual meaning'. He illustrates how language functions to conceal and distort the political elements intrinsic to the helping professions and how professional language serves to support and justify a hierarchy of power.

To summarize, specialist institutions – many of which may provide enriching and meaningful experiences for children – delineate children's space and organize their time, often within coercive contexts. They provide the foundation or the 'stage' on which rests a network of state-managed socializing activity. In this sense the benign institutional intentions expressed within professional discourse are subject to critique, and the political power of language comprises a key with which to understand its rhetorical constructions of reality. Central here, in terms of the processes of state socialization of children, is that specialist institutions regulate, reinforce and contain child–adult power relations within arrangements which claim to serve the 'best interests' of children. Further, the state has an established relation with the family which refines and complements on a micro-level such macro-level priorities.

The State–Family Relation: Production, Reproduction and the Processes of Social Replacement

So far, the above discussion has emphasized state regulation and the structural status of childhood. Within the advanced capitalist economies, however, a relation between the state and the family is forged within which obligations towards children, and the right to exercise authority and control over them, is negotiated and defined. The relation between the state and the family is both consensual, in the sense that the family is the preferred social institution to bear and to rear children, and contested, in that its form and its delineation is dynamic and shifts both in time and in space. As Shamgar-Handelman (1994:253) states, 'every element of this arrangement is always a subject for (overt, organised and legitimate, or covert and indirect) negotiation.' As the family fulfils an essential task, both in and for society, in bearing and raising children, so it occupies a special place and commands a level of institutional power. The state, through its network of institutional arrangements and bureaucratic organizations, accedes to the authority of the family, providing that it fulfils its socializing role satisfactorily and establishes a cordial and co-operative affiliation with state agencies and specialist institutions. The negotiating process is a manifestation of mutual dependence.

The power relations between the family and the state are invariably unequal and the cordiality of the relation will be determined largely by the compliance of the family and its considered suitability to raise children. Further, a striking feature of the negotiating process, whether it is located on the everyday primary level (as between parents and teachers), or at a higher institutional level (as in the case of High Court hearings), is the marginalization, if not total exclusion, of children (Donzelot, 1980; Freeman, 1983; Makrinioti, 1994; Shamgar-Handelman, 1994).

The state–family relation is determined by a duality of imperatives: the process of production and reproduction, and the processes of socialization and social replacement. The first comprises the domain of family planning and fertility policy, involving the regulation of the birth of (planned) children. Shamgar-Handelman notes:

> Be it an attempt to either increase or decrease the general number of members of the society in the next generation, the family is requested, tempted, pressured, or under a threat to oblige . . . In the main, it is social prestige and economic resources that are both offered and/or requested, and are used as rewards, as well as sanctions, in this process. The economic rewards granted to a family for complying with the requests of social [state] policy, or the economic sanctions for refraining from doing so, are usually specified in certain regulations or even in the law itself (1994:256).

The second, and complementary, element of the state–family relation is the transformative process within which children are expected to become suitable and acceptable future citizens. This duality of imperatives comprises the processes of physical replacement and social replacement. The family is the crucial institution in the realization of both imperatives and, in this sense, families 'own' children. Makrinioti observes:

childhood [is fused] into the family institution to such an extent that it becomes an inseparable unit, which obstructs the social visibility of its weaker part as a separate entity. Children by nature belong to their parents . . . children's social identity is seen to mirror that of their parents. The child is an open window to the family, and the family is portrayed in the child (1994:268).

Not all families, however, are considered as 'suitable' in the raising and socializing of children and herein lies the determination of family versus state ownership and control of childhood. Disproportionate numbers of working class, black, and lone parent families attract the gaze of state agencies and are exposed to state-directed family interventions, becoming targets of institutionalized scorn and blame (Dominelli, 1988; Dominelli and McLeod, 1989; Jones, 1983; Parton, 1985, 1991). It follows that the level, nature and source of adult power, the control and authority to which the child is subjected will be determined by adult professional judgments and assessments of the parenting capacities of adult family members. At the extremes, as Shamgar-Handelman (1994:261) observes, 'the state and/or authorized agencies have legal power to deny the right of some families to raise the children who were born to them, as it has the power to give families the right to bring up children that were not born to them.' Consequently children are treated as property and the custodianship of the property is determined by professional adjudication. Whether it is the interests of children or the priorities of the state which are negotiated during such interventions remains a fundamental issue for debate.

Childhood and Gender Relations: The Limitations and the Potential of Feminist Analyses

Thus far the theoretical analyses outlined tend to juxtapose the constructions of adulthood and childhood as if they are respectively homogenous and unified as structural categories. Although the concept of *childhoods* has been introduced, adulthood has been presented as a cognate, consistent and uniform category. Perhaps the most fundamental shortcoming of such an analysis is its agendered emphasis. Indeed, as Qvortrup notes:

Given the fact that women more often than men have taken care of children, that children historically were always a 'woman's business' much more than a male responsibility, there are good reasons for holding the view that one should really not speak in general terms about children's relationships with adults, but rather distinguish between women and men (1994:14).

Indeed, children's primary care is routinely and institutionally assigned to women in both the private domain (mother, housewife) and in the public domain (care-taking jobs). The relation of women and children is such that it requires a refined analysis which cannot be reduced solely to the adulthood–childhood relation. The fact that patriarchal social relations have institutionalized children as women's appendages or, conversely, women have been ascribed and largely confined within mothering and caring activity, has problematized and polarized the woman–child relation within much feminist analysis, treating women and children as adversaries. Alanen argues:

> feminist theory has not disrupted the sociological inheritance of marginalizing children; in discussing gender issues related to children, it has, unfortunately, remained just as functionalist and adult-centred in its analyses as mainstream/malestream social science (1994:34).

This indicates a fundamental limitation of many feminist analyses, in that its primary frame of reference is intrinsically adultist. Yet, feminist theorizing and enquiry also offers considerable potential in terms of its, as yet, largely under-developed contribution to a critical sociology of childhood. The structural commonality between the social location and positioning of women and children which, as Alanen (1994:35) notes, have been 'repeatedly mentioned since the beginning of feminist scholarship . . . may provide useful leads for rethinking the relationship between children and adults as being analogous to the relationship between men and women.' Also, analyses of locations in which gender relations and child–adult relations interface offer illuminating theoretical dimensions concerning the space and social reality of children. Concepts of 'otherness' and 'subject–object' dichotomy, as discussed earlier, central to feminist analyses are also significant in interpreting the structural position of children, offering a critique of dominant ideological constructions and pervasive social consciousness. For it is here that the child is defined and differentiated with reference to adults, not adults with reference to children. The deconstructionist direction of feminist theories, their fundamental critique of the ideological forms and images of women and feminity, have relevance not only to gendered, patriarchal relations between children but also to the structural relations of adultism. Further, many of the research techniques and methodological approaches developed within feminisms can be applied to a critical study of childhood (see, for example, Bell and Roberts, 1984:3; Finch, 1984:85; Harvey, 1990:104–11; Scraton, 1989:358; Stanley and Wise, 1983).

Childhood and Economic Relations: Generation and Poverty

Despite the child-welfare proclamations of government (see Department of Health, 1994) and the rhetorical constructions of national childcare intrinsic to liberal democracy, the structural and institutional exclusion and marginalization of childhood, the outsider status of children means that they are the age group most exposed to economic disadvantage (NCH Action for Children, 1995; Oppenheim, 1993; Sgritta, 1994). Although charities and campaigns regularly succeed in mobilizing national sentiment in order to 'give a child a chance', and are applauded for their 'good works', childhood has no chance in the sense of open opportunities within the context of economic relations. Children are entirely dependent on, and financially tied to, adults. They have no legitimate claim to income in their own right and their exclusion from state benefits has been extended in recent years compounding the dependency status of young people. Parents, then, are solely responsible for children's economic well-being and 'this ideological claim becomes much more problematic when we realize that children in terms of distributive justice do not fare particularly well at all' (Qvortrup, 1994:16).

The economics of childhood is a neglected area, but even the most cursory analysis of childhood and economic relations in Britain exposes a reality in stark contrast to the child welfare proclamations and rhetorical constructions of national childcare referred to earlier. Four point one million children in Britain, nearly 35 per cent of the population, live in families with incomes less than half the national average. This number has grown from 3.9 million in 1991–92 (NCH Action for Children, 1995:41) and black children particularly are disadvantaged (Joseph Rowntree Foundation, 1995). Children in over 750,000 families living on income support have deficient diets, and nearly 12,000 children under 16 years go hungry because there is insufficient money to buy food (NCH Action for Children, 1995:6). These statistics demonstrate the unequal distribution of income and wealth which is a universal reality of capitalist economies affecting children *and* adults. The point being, however, that children are excluded from economic rights in a society characterized by deepening and widening economic inequality (Joseph Rowntree Foundation, 1995). That children 'have no rights that are not mediated by the family' supports 'a system that has shown itself to be profoundly inadequate for guaranteeing justice between the generations' (Sgritta, 1994:358–9).

Conclusion

The primary purpose here has been to 'provoke a rethinking of settled ideas about children' and childhood (Scarre, 1989:x). It has been argued that it is necessary to dig below surface meaning and to interrogate dominant notions of *children* and *childhood* which are underpinned by *naturalistic* and biologically-determined conceptualizations. Childhood must be historically and theoretically contextualized, and the social, economic and political arrangements that determine its form require critical examination. The politics of childhood is central to this examination, being a politics consistently concerned with children's place: work, street, school, home. Historical constructions and reconstructions of childhood have relocated children from mill, mine and factory into school and family, and the contemporary debates are underpinned with rhetorical pronouncements regarding 'strengthening the family' as the 'basic unit of society', serving the 'best interests of the child' and 'developing the development of children'. In this sense children are objects for both care and control and what society does *to* them is profoundly confused with what society does *for* them. The otherness of children and the power relations which underpin the child–adult relation have to be unpacked. Childhood requires a conceptual autonomy within the contexts of intra-structural and inter-structural analysis. Children are not only future members *of* society they are active participants *within* society, and as such the temporal and spatial institutional arrangements intrinsic to familial and state forms of socialization require critical scrutiny. There is little time for complacency as western industrial states experience substantial structural changes. Bardy notes:

> The very foundations of societies – where childhood and adulthood are positioned – are open to new and, indeed, in many ways unknown developments. Extensive material and mental changes are 'pushing' societies and states towards new, major changes, involving the organization of labour, family structures, personal and collective ideals, renewed building of nations, and even the entire world (1994:316).

The coming generations of children no longer will grow up and go to school before entering the world of work within the same nationally bounded conditions that applied to their parents. Contemporary society already is strained by structured unemployment, deepening and widening polarization and pervasive inequality and injustice. Further construction and reconstruction of childhood is imminent in response to the profound challenges that lie within a foreboding socioeconomic and political context.

Chapter 2

'Crisis': The Demonization of Children and Young People

Howard Davis and Marc Bourhill

In February 1993 the abduction, suffering and murder of a 2-year-old boy on Merseyside became the symbol of a society in social and moral decline. As the blurred security video images of James Bulger, led through a busy shopping mall by two young boys, were broadcast around the world, media and political commentaries proclaimed that exceptional levels of violence within British society had been reached. Many explanations and numerous 'experts' fuelled the national debate, but two closely related assumptions prevailed: the decline of the family and parental discipline; the lost innocence of a previous 'golden age' of childhood. Since those images were first broadcast the *crisis in childhood* has been a persistent theme, dominating the press, broadcast news, features and documentaries. It has been the focus of parliamentary debates and official inquiries while also featuring in drama and television soaps. The media, particularly the press, have sustained the moral panic and political outrage, often stoking the fire with the latest burning revelation, regardless of the truth. Children and young people remain conspicuous by their absence in all but their misdeeds or as targets for (adult) popular judgment or academic analysis. This chapter critically assesses the form, content and implications of these developments, setting them in their contemporary contexts. It compares the recent coverage of children as perpetrators with that of the physical and sexual abuse of children within the family, the place where children are most at risk.

The Media, Social Construction and Childhood

Hall (1973:86) argues that news 'is a product, a human construction' created within social, political, economic and cultural contexts. From a mass of daily events the news is distilled, selected and presented (Cohen and Young, 1973; Glasgow Media Group, 1976, 1980, 1982). The processes of selection and presentation are underpinned by 'news values', shaped by what is deemed newsworthy (Hetherington, 1985; Tunstall, 1971). According to Coleman *et al.* (1990:8) 'the newsworthiness of events is based on an assumed set of news imperatives common to the genre'. Chibnall (1977) lists these imperatives as: immediacy; dramatization; personalization; simplification; titillation; conventionalism; novelty; structured access. Rock (1973:77) concludes that 'much news is, in fact, ritual . . . endlessly repeated drama whose themes are familiar and well understood.'

Journalists, trained with these news values and pressured by tight deadlines in a competitive arena, utilize well-established practices, particularly routinized contact with official institutions and 'expert' individuals. Most news, contrary to the popular image, is not the result of energetic journalists going in search of stories, but reflects an inflow of official information. Such officials, spokespersons, politicians, professionals and 'experts' become positioned as primary definers, establishing the framework within which social events and problems are presented and reconstructed. They set the agenda (Cohen and Young, 1973; Hall *et al.*, 1978). They enjoy privileged, structured access, which often leads to distortion and bias in the coverage. As Scraton, Jemphrey and Coleman state:

> This is not simply a matter of conspiracy theory. Journalists . . . are trained and employed in well-established and highly regulated practices which come to inform their news gathering activities. In a sense they apply a formula to their work, a 'vocabulary of precedence', closely related to the particular branch or form of media in which they work (1995:227).

The combination of the journalist's assimilation of news values, characterized by integrating sensationalism with conventionalism, and a dependence on the contributions of official agencies and experts, creates and sustains conformity in news presentation. Herman and Chomsky argue:

> Given the imperatives of corporate organization and the workings of various filters, conformity to the needs and interests of privileged sectors is essential to success. In the media, as in other major institutions, those who do not display the requisite values and perspectives will be regarded as 'irresponsible', 'ideological', or otherwise aberrant, and will tend to fall by the wayside. While there may be a small number of exceptions, the pattern is pervasive and expected. Those who adapt, perhaps quite honestly, will then be free to express themselves with little managerial control, and they will be able to assert, accurately, that they perceive no pressures to conform (1988:304).

The media portrayal of children's involvement in crime, either as perpetrators or victims, is central in creating and reinforcing public perceptions of childhood. While this has consequences for children, individually and collectively, its derivation lies within a broader context of media and political concern over a perceived breakdown in law and order. The role of the media in creating and sustaining moral panics reflective of such a breakdown has received substantial sociological attention. Cohen's definitive work on moral panics in the early

1970s maintains that their construction and persistence reflect a 'condition, episode, person or group' as constituting 'a threat to societal values or interests':

> its nature is presented in a stylized and stereotypical fashion by the mass media; the moral barricades are manned by editors, bishops, politicians and other right-thinking people; socially accredited experts pronounce their diagnoses and solutions; ways of coping are evolved or (more often) resorted to; the condition then disappears, submerges or deteriorates and becomes more visible (Cohen, 1973:9).

Golding and Middleton (1979) suggest three phases: the event which gives rise to the panic; a period in which previously latent mythologies about the constituted 'problem' emerge, and are debated; the government reaction to the concerns the media claims to be articulating on behalf of the public. As Hay argues, a model of moral panic does not imply that audiences are 'passive ideological dupes' as people receive information in the context of their lived realities and experiences: 'the moral panic thus becomes *lived* and begins to have substantive effects' (1995:198).

Given that moral panics have real consequences as they become mediated by authoritarian political rhetoric and state interventions, it is important to identify and examine 'latent mythologies' relevant to the assumed behaviour of children and young people. Central is the social construction of childhood, its relation to 'traditional' views of the family, and the exaltation and exploitation of the latter in appeals to 'common-sense' on law and order. As R. and W. Stainton-Rogers (1992:12) state, the ways 'children are construed not only determine the way we make sense of them as children, but also inform and reflect social and economic policies towards children and the institutions that manage children.'

In examining the key features of the modern, western construction of childhood, Archard (1993) identifies the significance of children's 'separateness' from adults – in their expected behaviour, their worlds and the expectations placed on them. It is not a separation of equals but, conversely, one which emphasizes inequality embodying incompetence and vulnerability. To be a child is to lack 'the capacities, skills and powers of adulthood'; to become an adult is to reject 'that which could never possibly serve the adult in the adult world' (1993:30). This developmental road to adulthood is mapped by adult, professional experts who manage the process of children becoming adults, providing directives and classifying the 'functional' and the 'dysfunctional'. Despite claims for objectivity and scientific method, the process is not value-free. It is bound to theoretical and sub-theoretical conceptions determined by and determining of the adult norm. For Piaget the state of maturity was the capacity for abstract and hypothetical thinking, and for Freud it was the attainment of a genital, heterosexual desire (Archard, 1993:33). Yet powerful and clearly defined assumptions permeate popular beliefs about how adults and children differ (R. and W. Stainton-Rogers, 1992). At the heart of western belief systems, and deeply-rooted in the British tradition, are stereotypes founded on binary opposites: innocence v. evil; nature v. nurture; protection v. freedom.

Media treatment of issues about children relies heavily on such simplistic generalizations with children represented as objects of concern or as threats to adult order. The former relies on an idealized view of children as pure, innocent and vulnerable, needing protection or salvation from dangers they can neither identify nor comprehend. The latter, of children drawn innately (unless prevented) towards evil and anarchy, also has deep historical roots (Miller, 1983). It is a portrayal powerfully evoked by William Golding's (1959) novel, *Lord of the Flies*. The power of this fictional work is evident in the frequency with which it is given respect and credibility in press accounts of 'deviant' children. It evokes an apocalyptic vision of anarchy as being inevitable should children lose the discipline and order of the adult presence. R. and W. Stainton-Rogers (1992:191) conclude that the portrayals of children as 'innocent victims' or 'culpable delinquents' are no more than 'alternative placements that the adult world creates . . . into which children are located at different times, in different circumstances.' The idea that children are products of nature or nurture leads to media concern as to whether child 'deviance' is rooted in a biological predisposition or in an environmental determinism. Children's meanings and motivations are persistently ignored, as is the position of adults, both familial and professional, as powerful definers of deviant behaviour. Consequently, much of the physical and psychological harm inflicted on children by adults is disregarded, while transgressions by children of their set role are the subject of furious condemnation.

The circumstances which contextualize moral panics are substantially affected by the prevailing political climate. The election of the Conservatives under the Thatcherite, New Right agenda in 1979, which delivered the pre-election promises of social authoritarianism, transformed the political, economic and social landscape. Closely related to the ascribed 'crisis' in law and order (rising crime, militant unions, declining moral standards, street demonstrations) was the powerful rhetoric concerning the decline of the family. As the free-market economy impacted in socially divisive ways, state authoritarianism demanded legitimation (Hall *et al.*, 1978; Scraton, 1987). The 'enemies within' were many: 'muggers', miners, trade-unionists, 'loony-left' councils, immigrants, travellers, youths and, most recently, the homeless, single parents and their children. Those most affected by mass unemployment and impoverishment have been those consigned to the social margins, condemned roundly for their own misfortune. Crime, lawlessness and disorder have been portrayed as illustrative of a decline in traditional values with children and young people depicted as bereft of personal responsibility, not knowing right from wrong and ill-disciplined due to the absence of effective punishment. The family and the school, along with youth justice reform, have been targeted as responsible for this disciplinary decline.

From the early 1980s the New Right idealized the traditional family, 'not a million miles away from the White Anglo-Saxon Protestant (model)' (Frost, 1990:35). This portrayal marginalized those not fitting the ideal. As Parton explains:

> while stressing the need for a reduced state, [this position] requires a strong state to establish certain modes of family life . . . It has at its root an individualized conception of social relations whereby the market is the key institution for the economic sphere, while the family is the key institution for the social sphere (1991:202).

Thus the burden of providing appropriate and necessary services was removed from the tax payer as social responsibility and is placed on 'failing families' as individual responsibility. Within the context of this shift crimes committed by children have acquired new significance.

Children as Criminals

> The 1979 Thatcher Administration not only repoliticised crime and punishment but dramatised it to the point where it came to assume an importance in the political bestiary akin to that previously only granted to the Warsaw Pact and the National Union of Mineworkers (Pitts, 1988:43).

The fear of youth crime and lawlessness is not new and Pearson (1983) demonstrates that every British generation has experienced 'hooligans' alongside nostalgic claims for a past 'golden age' free of such threats. In the 1960s it was 'mods and rockers' (Cohen, 1973); previously it was 'Teddy boys'. Pearson shows similar concerns with the original, Victorian 'hooligans', ironically a period identified by the New Right as exemplifying order and discipline through Victorian values (see also Sindall, 1990). Within this context stories of youth crime are frequent, and regularly juxtaposed and conflated with extraordinary or bizarre aspects of youth culture (Muncie, 1984:13). Crimes committed (or alleged) by children, although more rare, offer greater potential for sensationalism and in their reports newspapers commonly highlight the real or estimated ages of the youngest 'involved'.

A typical example appeared in the *Daily Mirror* (7 August 1991) which reported an attack on a man whose face was slashed. Alongside his photograph was the headline: 'Slashed . . . For Asking Yobs To Keep Quiet So His Grandchildren Could Sleep'. The perpetrators were depicted as 'yobs', impersonal outsiders, in contrast to the respectable 'insider', an ordinary grandfather merely requesting consideration for his family. The story did not explore motives but reported that the 'gang of thugs' included 'some as young as NINE'. In alleging the participation of such young children in such a demonstrable act of serious violence the report challenged popular assumptions of childhood innocence. Such actions were presented as evidence that the fabric of society was crumbling. The *Daily Mirror* sought opinion from an 'expert' on 'sick children in gangs', suggesting that such violence constituted evidence of mental illness. The report signified the relationship between individual and social pathology. Yet the two youths who were charged were aged 17 and 18, raising doubts about the younger children being active participants. The brief reference, made the following day, concerning a visit by the 'shocked kids' who had been present, was a clear indication that they were no more than bystanders who witnessed the attack (*Daily Mirror*, 8 August 1991). In fact, the involvement of young children in serious crime is rare. Yet during 'moral panics' such cases are actively sought out, exaggerated or invented. For example, in February 1993, at the time of the James Bulger murder, much coverage was given to 'rat-boy', a young person occupying the recesses and roof spaces of a housing complex and the meter cupboards lined with bits of carpet. He was accused of terrorizing an entire estate (*Daily Mail*, 27 February 1993).

Occasionally, such elaboration extends beyond an individual child to groups or communities of 'criminals' with stories exaggerated and mythologized. In 1982 such a story broke in Liverpool, at St Saviours School, Toxteth, leading to the Prime Minister, Margaret Thatcher, making a statement to the House of Commons. The *Daily Star* (23 February 1982) announced a 'Rampage of Tiny Terrors', in which a 'mini-mafia' allegedly: 'covered cars in kitchen swill'; 'soaked teachers with extinguishers'; 'slashed furniture with knives'; 'set fire to their books'. Further, it was claimed that they tore down ceiling tiles, and 'ransacked classrooms'. The *Daily Mirror* (23 February 1982) also carried the story: 'Mini Mobsters School Terror'. The *Daily Mail* (23 February 1982) repeated the allegations but located the 'orgy of violence and destruction' within the context of 'provocation by left-wing extremists'. A 'primary definer', City Councillor Michael Storey was quoted extensively as claiming that 'militant groups' had leafleted the children in 'a deliberate attempt to stir up hatred' (*Daily Mail*, 23 February 1982).

The *Daily Mail*, ironically for a paper committed to the efficacy of corporal punishment, reported Storey's deputy, Ann Clitheroe, as lamenting, 'Last week Mr McLoughlin (the headteacher) caned seven pupils. An hour later fourteen windows were smashed.' The following day the media identified the 'ringleader' of its mini-mafia: 'Girl of Ten Led Gang Terror' (*Daily Mirror*, 24 February 1982). The inside headline was: 'Little Miss Mobster'. The girl was described as an extortionist, an arsonist and a tearaway. The *Daily Star* (24 February 1982) described her as 'big, black and really nasty'. Subsequently, *The Sunday Times* (28 February 1982) contradicted this public character assassination of a 10-year-old, quoting school reports in her defence and describing her as 'bright' and 'highly imaginative'. It was too late, the media had mobilized a powerful symbol: a girl, black, from Toxteth and just 10 years old. While the girl's mother defended her daughter against this vicious attack (*Daily Mirror*, 25 February 1982), the damage was done and St Saviours became synonymous with a 'crisis in schools' indicative of national breakdown. The *Daily Mail* leader (24 February 1982) entitled 'The little savages of St Saviour's [*sic*]' combined child-hating language, apocalyptic imagery and reactionary, punitive portrayal:

> It reads like the script of a futuristic horror movie . . . If children of 8 to 10 can intimidate adults supposed to be in authority over them, then are not the very foundations of our society giving way? . . . There is nothing either new or particular to the polyglot problem areas of inner cities about the inherent cruelty of young children.
>
> Remember *Lord of the Flies* . . . Original sin is what Golding was writing about . . . a religious concept, we suspect more relevant to the mayhem that occurred at this C of E school in Liverpool than any glib sociological generalisation. Children will run wild, viciously wild, unless they are properly supervised. They need parents to give them a stable and ordered home. They need teachers who know how to keep order as well as how to impart knowledge. They need, God help them, practical instruction in the difference between right and wrong (*Daily Mail*, 24 February 1982).

Here was a rhetoric established and developed which was to re-emerge throughout the next decade, particularly following the murder of James Bulger. It invoked Golding's construct of anarchy inherent in children left to themselves.

However, the 'causes' of the problem lie not just with inherently deviant children but in the supposed subversion of those institutions that are supposed to constrain this deviance – in the 'trendy' progressivism of schools and other institutions, and the 'breakdown' of 'family values'. Two days after its leader, the *Daily Mail* commented on a European Court ruling against physical punishment to children without their parents' permission (hardly progressive given that it was grounded in the rights of parents, not children):

> It is ironical that the Strasbourg Court of Human Rights has pronounced against corporal punishment in our schools just after the terrible infant violence which caused St Saviour's [*sic*] infant school in Toxteth to be closed. This hardly seems a time for removing restraints. Yet they seem to have managed for years on the Continent without the cane, and with less vandalism. Perhaps their secret is that, unlike ourselves, they have kept clear of trendy methods of modern education and clung to the traditional structural approach,

so the children are more absorbed in their work and less liable to run wild (*Daily Mail*, 26 February 1982).

What the story of St Saviours demonstrates is that the press uses a pre-defined template in the framing of such stories. What is absent in the account (children's versions, children's rights issues, marginalization, critical examinations of the 'traditional family') is as important as what is present (calls for more discipline, deviant families or groups, subversion of 'traditional' values and institutions). Such alleged crimes are often wildly exaggerated (in the case of St Saviours the allegations were rejected by a full inquiry) in terms of their actuality and their significance, and amplified as part of a wider moral panic about crime and social indiscipline.

Children as Victims: The Media and Child Abuse

Since Rousseau's *Emile*, the image of the innocent and vulnerable child has been powerful (R. and W. Stainton-Rogers, 1992). Its construction and representation within the media, from news to features, from documentary to drama, is complex. Nowhere is this more evident than in recent coverage of physical, sexual and psychological child abuse. The mid-1980s was a period when the media discovered child abuse, and TV soaps, police dramas and other entertainment began to carry story-lines with childhood abuse often used as a simplistic explanation for any adult crime or deviation. Yet again, there were no shortage of 'experts', from those on BBC2's *Newsnight* to, more recently, Fitz as the morose, alcoholic, gambling psychologist in ITV's award-winning 1990s series, *Cracker*. Yet, for a media run by adults for their peers' consumption, the presentation of issues of child abuse as crime has posed significant difficulties.

Physical Abuse

Since the early 1970s, media coverage of a tragic succession of murders of children by their parents or caregivers have provided evidence that such events make 'good copy' (Franklin and Parton, 1991). The deaths of Maria Colwell in 1973, Jasmine Beckford in 1985 and Kimberly Carlile and Tyra Henry in 1987 at the hands of parents and step-parents were given considerable media attention. The faces of these children, staring out from tabloid front pages and social work textbooks remain imprinted in the minds of public and professional alike. These murders were projected as events of considerable broader significance, constituting a process of discovery, possibly rediscovery, of the abuse and murder of children by their parents or caregivers. The level and style of the publicity given to physical abuse, particularly those cases which result in death, was unprecedented. The extensive inquiries into recent deaths focused media attention on, and gave impetus to, rising rates of child abuse referrals and professional discourses seeking to publicize, explain and offer responses to 'the problem'. This discovery, and the tragedies which are its markers, has not been without political significance. Throughout this period the constitution and role of 'the family', and its relationship to the state, consolidated as central themes, reflecting critical and feminist discourses and, conversely, the hegemonic project of the New Right.

Responding to the newsworthiness of the murder and physical abuse of children has presented the news media with difficulties. 'Crime' stories tend to be reported, implicitly or explicitly, as part of the bigger story of a society 'in decline', a society in which 'traditional' values and institutions are collapsing. This bigger story depicts the crisis in law and order as rooted in declining traditional family values and the replacement of 'common-sense' punitive responses to crime by 'soft', 'trendy' and 'permissive' approaches mobilized by a subversive ideology of misplaced liberalism. Single parents, lack of self-reliance and dependency on the state, together with inadequate discipline, are persistent constructs underpinning the 'causes' of crime. This rhetoric has demanded the reaffirmation of punishment as both deterrent and retribution. The severe, or fatal physical assault on children by adults within the family is not easily accommodated within such a framework. How does physical abuse fit with demands for more, rather than less, punishment? In the private domain of the family, where is the line drawn between 'abuse' and 'punishment' (see Newell, 1989)? This dilemma has been resolved within the media by the pathologization of 'failed' or 'deviant' families. Family 'dysfunction' dovetails neatly with the representations of a breakdown in discipline and order. Yet it bears no relation to the reality of violence towards children which cannot be restricted to a few 'deviant' families.

Recalling the 'law and order' crisis of the 1970s (see Hall *et al.* 1978), Parton argues that 'the category of "violence" is both potentially all-encompassing and ideologically very powerful.' He continues:

> it is difficult to argue against it. This is particularly so when the victim is seen as 'innocent', as in the case of children. The case of Maria Colwell provided a focus for the expression of a range of social anxieties concerned with the collapse of the 'English way of life', the growth in violence, the decline in individual and social discipline and morality, and the need to re-establish the traditional family (1985:81).

While such anxieties are mobilized and reflected in media responses to reporting the physical abuse of children, they focus only on these 'problem' families and the scale of violence against children across society is not reflected. Most physical assaults on children are never reported as 'crime' and most perpetrated by parents are not defined as abusive. Uniquely among oppressed groups, children are not protected by law unless the assault is judged to go beyond 'reasonable' chastisement, usually meaning causing serious physical injury. As most physical abuse occurs in the privacy of the family home, it remains invisible. Instances known to outside agencies often do not result in prosecution as they are referred to closed case conferences, or are heard before the family court. Finally, a bruise sustained by a child from a violent parent, should it ever reach the attention of the media, would be classified as less newsworthy than a similar injury sustained in the street, or inflicted on an adult (particularly an older person) by a child or young person. The infliction of violence on children by adults is not news unless it is 'excessive', and therefore viewed as exceptional or an aberration. And it is underwritten by nostalgic calls for 'clips around the ear' which 'never did "us" any harm'.

As it is highly selective in its coverage of the murder and brutalization of children, the media reports only spectacular or exceptional cases, emphasizing those instances which occur outside the family. When children are killed within the family, the cases are often treated as routine. On the same page of the *Daily Mail* (19 August 1987) that a 14 paragraph piece headlined 'The Woman Who Failed Tragic Tyra' appeared, criticizing Tyra Henry's social worker, another story headed 'Father Who Killed His Baby Jailed For Life' was reported. It was given three sentences. Similarly, some days previously, under the heading 'Child Killer Jailed', the *Daily Mail* (8 December 1987) reported:

Sadistic Terry Langridge, 23, was jailed for ten years at Lewes in Sussex yesterday for kicking to death his lover's daughter, three year old Leanne. Her mother, Melanie Pelling, 27 from Brighton was given 18 months for neglect.

This was the piece in its entirety – two sentences long. It contrasts with the detailed coverage given to abductions, sex crimes and child killings outside the family, and child killings within, as part of suicide pacts. Examples of the former include: 'The Hostage: Muggers Hold Baby Girl At Knifepoint And Demand Cash' (*Daily Mail*, 23 February 1982); 'Girl, 6, Is Abducted In Beer Garden' (*Daily Express*, 7 August 1990); 'Beast Rapes Girl, 11, In Crowded Holiday Park' (*Daily Mirror*, 6 August 1991). Examples of the latter include: 'Wife And Her Lover Kill Children In Suicide Pact' (*Daily Express*, 1 August 1990); 'Toddler Sees Mother Shot Dead By Ex-Lover' (*Daily Express*, 7 August 1990). Yet, despite the frequency of such stories, a catalogue of abduction and mistreatment of children by adults, no moral panic is constructed. They are not accompanied by anguished media pronouncements warning of the collapse of society.

It is within this broader context of the invisibility of routine adult violence towards children that specific serious cases, often resulting in death, and usually involving social workers' failings, are reported widely and individualized. This individualized focus on 'deviant' families reflects and reinforces the official responses to child protection, particularly concerning violence and death (Loney, 1989; Parton, 1985). Consequently, social factors, material or cultural, are ignored. Indeed, in the media coverage of the Beckford, Carlile and Henry cases, little consideration was given to the fundamental question of why particular adults killed particular children. The *Daily Mirror* (30 March 1985) dealt with this briefly following the conviction of Maurice Beckford for the manslaughter of his stepdaughter, Jasmine, revealing that as a child he had been beaten with a tawse and locked in a shed by his father. But the report failed to develop the theme of parental violence as rooted in childhood experiences and its implications in a parentally violent society. Its main focus, typically, was the castigation of the social worker for having this information on file, but only seeing Jasmine once in ten months.

The simplistic reductionism in the coverage of such cases is evident in the typically pejorative adjectives used to describe the killer with little attention given to the context of the crime. Maurice Beckford was 'Merciless and Remorseless' (*Daily Mail*, 29 March 1985); Nigel Hall, who killed Kimberley Carlile was a 'Torturer' (*Daily Mirror*, 16 May 1987) and 'Arrogant and Brutal' (*Daily Mail*, 16 May 1987). Such labels limit knowledge of the crime, its context or its perpetrator. The place of families within the broader social structure, and the vulnerability of children within the family, remain neglected areas of consideration. In contrast, the killing of James Bulger led to an all-pervasive public examination of a 'crisis' in childhood. There is no comparative analysis applied to adults. The issue becomes individualized. As Loney states:

> A number of consequences flow from this particular construction of child abuse. The depiction of child abuse as an outcome of the 'sick' behaviour of a small number of individuals and families implies the need for skilled professionals to help those at risk. When intervention fails to protect a child, the assumption is that this is because the professionals are not doing their jobs properly ... Not only is its prevalence limited by the fact that it is only 'problem families' who pose a risk, but by making the prevention of further abuse a 'professional task', the rest of us are 'let off the hook' (1989:88).

This has led to 'the regular collective character assassination of social workers' (Golding, 1991:89). The press has been unequivocal in explaining the recurrent deaths of children in families: incompetent, naive, leftist social workers failing to protect children by leaving them with their obviously 'sick' or 'evil' parents.

The conviction of Maurice Beckford brought the front page banner headline in the *Daily Mirror* (29 March 1985): 'Jasmine Outrage'. It continued, 'Why was she taken from foster parents? Why was she only seen once in ten months? Why did the jury clear stepfather of murder?' The news coverage was similar, quoting Conservative MP Geoffrey Dickens as stating that the social workers' 'failure to detect the cruelty' was a 'scandal which defies comprehension'. The *Daily Mail's* headline was: 'Beyond Belief!', followed by a full page interview with Jasmine's foster parents entitled 'Torn from Love' (29 March 1985). The story ignored the acts that killed Jasmine, focusing on the response of Social Services. Photographs of Maurice Beckford and Beverley Lorrington (Jasmine's mother), were placed alongside photographs of Social Services' Assistant Director, 'Boss Simpson', with the caption, 'Hands in Pockets' (the judge had reprimanded him in court for having his hands in his pockets). In referring to the social worker it headlined 'Visitor Wahlstrom' with the caption, ' "Naive," said Judge.' After publication of the inquiry report the *Daily Mail* (3 December 1995) headlined its front-page story: 'Will No-One Take The Blame?' Its editorial asked, 'The man who killed Jasmine Beckford is where he ought to be . . . in prison serving his ten year sentence. But what of those who, if they had been doing their professional duty, could have averted this tragedy?'

This formula was repeated in the case of Kimberley Carlile. Following the trial verdict, the *Daily Mirror's* (16 May 1987) headline was 'How Did It Happen Again?' The report concluded that while the 'man who killed her' and 'her mother who did little to stop him' had been sentenced, 'others share in their guilt'. The 'problem' centred on social workers. As Franklin and Parton state:

> What is quite remarkable about media reporting of these three cases [Jasmine Beckford, Tyra Henry and Kimberley Carlile] of physical abuse, although the media present the matter as unexceptional and uncontentious, is their assumption that social workers should be considered as guilty for the death of the abused child as the abuser (1991:17).

Franklin and Parton argue that the vilification of social work as a profession is rooted in a number of factors. The focus on social workers involved in child deaths has not been merely a device to ignore the question of parental power, the continuum of violence against children and dangers of the adultist, patriarchal family. Social workers also have acted as a metaphor for the public sector as a whole. As a profession without roots or communally respected expertise, founded in legislation rather than tradition, it has provided an easy target. This is evident in the following two extracts:

> To what extent were the social workers of Brent 'naive' and to what extent were they blinded by dogma? What influence, if any did colour have on the disastrous decisions they took . . . Is there something wrong with their training; something in the agit-prop atmosphere of the inner-cities; something in the unfeeling arrogance of local bureaucracy that can dull the intelligence and humanity of the social worker? (*Daily Mail*, 29 March 1995).

> Indeed this case prompts the thought that if there were no social workers, the whole community would be more vigilant and responsi-

ble ... The trouble with today's Britain is that we have nationalised compassion and are pained when we discover what we should have known – that nationalised industries don't always care (*Daily Mail*, 6 May 1987).

In seeking to solve the problem, all newspapers accepted successive inquiry calls for better management of child abuse cases and improved training, but their scepticism about social work as a profession is well illustrated in the following *Daily Telegraph* (4 December 1985) response:

In the matter of field work, too much has been made of training, too little of experience and maturity. Poor Miss Wahlstrom, who is not a public enemy and must not be turned into an alibi, made mistakes which a middle-aged woman with her own children would not have made. How ready are the authorities to make intelligent use of middle-aged female common sense recruited late and not much burdened by sociology courses.

Rather than confront the real difficulties in managing the contradictions of intervening for the child while respecting the rights of parents and family autonomy in a climate of swingeing cuts and service reduction, it has proved easier for politicians and media to ridicule those whose professional judgment was found wanting (Franklin and Parton, 1991). For those suffering such public vilification, the consequences are profound (Ruddock, 1991).

The physical abuse of children by adults has been presented in a form which minimizes the implications for traditional and New Right views of the family, and adult/child relations. Popular discourse, supported by political commentaries, have associated pathological families with ideologically-motivated social workers, harnessing the emotive power of the image of the innocent and vulnerable child in the service of a broader, reactionary political project. By blaming pathological, 'inadequate' or dysfunctional families and subversive, poorly-trained social workers, a more searching and contextualizing examination of the physical abuse of children by adults is avoided. Unlike the general treatment of 'crime', crimes against children by parents and carers are one category of crime minimized by the media. Rather than identifying the possible links between these child deaths and broader issues such as structural inequality and the widespread, socially sanctioned use of violence against children, these are represented as the crimes of a deviant minority against their unfortunate, vulnerable children.

Sexual Abuse and Cleveland

As with physical abuse, the sexual abuse of children is not a recent phenomenon but it is well established in professional discourses (Rush, 1980). In the late nineteenth century Freud recorded the childhood 'seductions' of his female patients (Masson, 1984) but refuted these accounts, describing them as fantasies. The reality of the suffering was buried, neglected by the emerging professions of psychology and psychiatry, and hidden from wider debate (Masson, 1984, 1992; Miller, 1985). The rediscovery of child sexual abuse was not a result of an investigative and enlightened media but developed through the work and experiences of feminists and child protection practitioners. Feminist critiques and research addressed sexual abuse, particularly of girl children, in the context of sexual assault and violence against women. Child protection workers, through their surveillance of children at risk within their families, dealt daily with the consequences of the endemic abuse of children.

During the 1980s, however, sexual abuse became increasingly newsworthy, promoted through coverage by television social issues presenter Esther Rantzen. She was influential in launching Childline, a helpline for children. The coverage emphasized children as the innocent victims of specifically male predatory behaviour. As R. and W. Stainton-Rogers (1992:28) point out, however, it is precisely the attribution of 'innocence' to childhood that 'makes children . . . targets for those for whom the corrupting potential of sex is a key to gaining sexual release.' Further, as Kitzinger (1988:80) argues, 'innocence' is a 'suspect concept' because it 'stigmatises the "knowing" child'. The portrayal of 'innocence', however, became the powerful image central to coverage of child sexual abuse, delivering the message that it was not an aberration but a frequent occurrence in many families.

The emergent research challenged the myth that abuse was restricted to a 'type' of easily pathologized family, but indicated that sexual abuse cut across class boundaries (Finkelhor, 1986). Unlike physical abuse, the perpetrators of sexual abuse were, overwhelmingly, men (see Finkelhor, 1986; Herman, 1981; Macleod and Saraga, 1988). Further, they were men who appeared to be 'normal'. As the story unfolded, women with children were faced with the possibility that their partners could be sexually abusing their children. Non-abusing men were faced with the reality that many of their gender, from whom they could not be easily differentiated, were sexual abusers. Further, many parents held secrets concerning their own childhood experiences. The presentation of sexual abuse, unlike that of physical abuse, carried possible implications and profound anxieties for 'our' family and not just others.

The acceptance of widespread child sexual abuse demanded a reappraisal of children's experiences and a fresh interpretation of children's behaviour and play. Children, previously 'seen but not heard', required close attention. Although not usually fatal, sexual abuse was often a more shocking discovery than physical abuse. While adults supporting chastisement and physical punishment as part of the context of 'discipline' might have been occasionally sympathetic to those who used 'excessive' violence 'in desperation', there was much less tolerance of child sexual abuse. It constituted a discovery potentially more subversive of traditional adultist and patriarchal beliefs about the family than did physical abuse. The collective anxiety subsequently generated was evident in the media attention it received; this was the prevailing climate when events in Cleveland hit the headlines.

The *Daily Mail* (20 June 1987), crusading on behalf of 'innocent' parents, broke the story with a front-page banner headline, claiming that Cleveland Council had ordered parents of 200 youngsters to 'Hand Over Your Child'. According to the newspaper such demands, supported by Court orders, occurred after routine visits to hospital. 'Cleveland', the place firmly synonymous with the case (Cream, 1993), was precipitated by a dramatic increase in the number of children diagnosed as sexually abused, and consequently removed from their families. Campbell comments on the procedures for managing child sexual abuse referrals as they operated at the time:

> An entire juggernaut is set into motion which historically has been based on child torture and battering. Sexual abuse was stuck in a framework concerned with acts that might end a child's life rather than acts which might ruin it . . . When the Cleveland crisis erupted, the procedures in most areas of the country were not modified to manage the entirely different dilemmas thrown up by sexual abuse (1988:7).

Nava (1988) distinguishes two phases in the intense media focus on Cleveland. First, was confusion which mirrored the range of positions taken by 'experts' as to prevalence, diagnosis and implications of sexual abuse. An example of this was a reflective and relatively balanced feature in the *Daily Telegraph* (25 June 1987) entitled 'Children at Risk: the Agonising Dilemma'. Even the *Daily Mail* did not reject the existence or significance of sexual abuse. Prior to breaking the Cleveland story, it gave prominent coverage to the subject, although focusing on sexual assault *outside* the family. A main feature exposed a paedophile ring in Holland in which '70 [children] are brutalised and paying the price of porn liberation' (*Daily Mail*, 12 June 1987). Other headlines included: 'Freed to Rape Girls 29 Times' (*Daily Mail*, 17 June 1987); 'Rape in the Infant School' (*Daily Mail*, 19 June 1987); 'Don't Shield the Monster Who Raped My Child' (*Daily Mail*, 20 June 1987).

Over Cleveland, however, the *Daily Mail* had no doubt as to the victims: the 'innocent' parents. Relying heavily on parents' versions, it ran the headline 'Victims of the Abuse Experts', subtitled, 'The Continuing Nightmare of Innocent Parents Who Stand Accused'. What was problematic was accepting that sexual abuse might have occurred in respectable, middle-class families: 'all involve educated, middle-class people who opened their doors freely to the professionals, believing they had nothing to fear' (*Daily Mail*, 24 June 1987). The following day the paper ran the headline 'These Innocent Parents' (*Daily Mail*, 25 June 1987) giving prominence to experts on the side of the parents, notably Dr Raine Roberts, a Manchester Police surgeon. Ironically, a year later the *Daily Mail* (7 July 1988) noted that her intervention was criticized in the subsequent inquiry report as being 'far from neutral'.

Nava (1988:115–18) argues that a process of personalization and polarization occurred, portraying female professionals alleging sexual abuse set against a range of male professionals and politicians 'on the side of the families'. This was fuelled by the allegations made by Stuart Bell MP (1988), and later refuted by the inquiry (Butler-Sloss, 1988:166), but at that time reported on the *Daily Mail's* (30 June 1987) front page under the headline: 'The Conspiracy'. Photographs of Dr Marietta Higgs, Consultant Paediatrician, and Susan Richardson, Social Services Child Abuse Consultant, accompanied the article, each with the caption 'Accused'. Other newspapers were not so quick to condemn Higgs and Richardson. Early in July articles appeared which emphasized concerns over sexual abuse, drawing on the views of Esther Rantzen, Valerie Howarth (Director of Childline) and Michelle Elliott (author of *Kidscape*). Their responses were supportive of Higgs, and covered widely (*Daily Telegraph*, 1 July 1987; *Sunday Mirror*, 28 July 1987; *Sunday Times*, 5 July 1987).

While Cleveland posed problems for journalists, particularly as 'experts' were polarized on the issues, of concern was the speed and apparent ease with which some newspapers did feel able to rush to judgments. For example, *The Independent* (30 June 1987) carried the following editorial:

> Social changes have made both sexual abuse, and the inclination to discover such abuse where it does not exist, more likely. Divorce, remarriage and the increasing acceptance of illegitimacy means that growing numbers of children live with a step-parent ... forms of sexual activity which were, until recently, considered deviant have become commonplace ... Further, militant feminists are inclined to consider all men sexually aggressive and rapacious until proved innocent. The nuclear family, once the highest ideal, is now too often regarded as unnatural and unattractive ... There is a danger that fashionable prejudice ... [will] label parents guilty until proved innocent and break up families before rather than after abuse has been confirmed (quoted in Nava, 1988:118).

Unable to accommodate sexual abuse within traditional assumptions of the idealized family this linked fashionable ideas about sexual abuse with 'deviant' and 'dangerous' sexual politics. Sexual abuse existed, but its prevalence was wildly exaggerated by some doctors and social workers who were over-zealous and 'authoritarian'.

The complex and detailed findings of the Inquiry, a year later, further exposed the intentions of newspapers with different agendas. The *Guardian* (7 July 1988) provided a detailed and thoughtful leading article covering the confirmation of the prevalence and the intrafamilial gendered nature of sexual abuse, the significance of signs of anal dilatation for diagnosis, and the proposed legal and procedural changes. In contrast, the *Daily Mail* (7 July 1988). remained steadfast. It asked, 'Who was to blame?' and 'How was it in those five terrible months that so much needless suffering could be inflicted on so many families in Cleveland?' In its central feature it acknowledged that the Report seriously criticized some of those with whom it had been closely associated over the previous year. Yet only a passing reference was made to the inaccurate and misleading information contained in Stuart Bell's dossier, on which the newspaper had relied and had conferred unquestioning legitimacy. Instead, under the front page headline, 'Not One Sign Of Regret', the *Daily Mail* continued its familiar, personalized focus on Dr Higgs, her colleague Dr Wyatt, Sue Richardson and Social Services Director Michael Bishop. It concluded, 'however "even-handed" the Report . . . Ministers believe these four must take the main blame for the collective hysteria that many shattered families will never forgive or forget' (*Daily Mail*, 7 July 1988). Similarly, the *Daily Mirror* (7 July 1988) captioned photographs of Higgs, Wyatt and Richardson as 'Guilty', and above the headline 'Never Again', implicitly criticized the Report, 'Doctors Under Fire in Cleveland Child Sexual Storm but Innocent Parents Aren't Cleared'. This theme dominated reporting, headlining another column: 'Anguish of the tragic parents'.

The conclusion to the Cleveland 'crisis' was ambivalent. Professionals, including doctors, police officers and social workers were criticized, but sexual abuse was confirmed as widespread and 'innocence' was not ascribed to all the parents in this particular episode. The personalized focus on professional mismanagement, however, rather than on the social and cultural roots of male abusive behaviour, allowed the media to accept the existence of abuse, while expressing scepticism over its prevalence and pouring scorn on the handling of allegations. Subsequently, media treatment of 'innocent' parents and 'incompetent', 'authoritarian' social workers after further 'crises' in Orkney and Rochdale confirmed this position. The complexities of child sexual abuse were brushed aside. Indeed, persistent media denial of the prevalence of sexual abuse went beyond the condemnation of professionals, as older myths of children as vindictive liars or as having 'false memories' were reasserted. As Nigel de Gruchy (quoted in the *Guardian*, 16 March 1994), general secretary of the NASUWT teaching union put it, 'Children are much more sexually aware than they ever were, and they're looking for things, and they know that if they can make an accusation then they can make the teacher pay for it, even if the accusation is totally false and malicious – and the majority of such accusations are.'

The sexual abuse of children is seen quite differently from other crime. Its prevalence is minimized, its 'causes' are scarcely discussed. Those engaged in 'the fight against' this particular crime are undermined, condemned and ridiculed. The 'folk devil' is not the abuser within the family, but the social workers or doctor deemed to have acted improperly. Or, as de Gruchy exemplifies, it is a lying, 'malicious' child.

James Bulger: From Murder to 'Childhood in Crisis'

Whatever the strength of the obsessive media coverage of 'persistent young offenders' and the political capital made from the 'breakdown of the family' debate in the build up to the 1992 General Election, what happened early in 1993 overshadowed all that had gone before. In February the tragic abduction and murder of 2-year-old James Bulger by two 10-year-old boys unleashed a moral outrage unprecedented in its emotive force. The case and its aftermath was a tragedy of international proportions. There are several reasons why this particular moral panic was quite so powerful. First was how the crime was represented in terms of traditional images and understanding of childhood as equating with 'innocence'. As Hay points out, this was not straightforward, because central to the power of the panic was that both the killers and the victim were children:

> For ten-year-old children tend to feature in mediated crime reporting as idealized innocent victims in relation to which the deviancy of the 'other' is defined. Here such conventional assumptions become challenged and this gives the Bulger case a much greater societal purchase, as we [the viewer, the reader] are effectively confronted by the implications of the realisation that those *formerly* conceived of as innocent victims might pose a profound threat themselves (1995:200–1).

The shock value of the crime was related to its rarity, a point occasionally noted in media coverage. Melanie Phillips and Martin Kettle reported (*Guardian*, 16 February 1993) that in 1991, 74 under-fives were murdered, none killed by strangers. Over the previous ten years only one child under five each year was killed by a stranger, with the exception of 1987 (three) and 1983 and 1991 (none). The James Bulger murder was an exception, yet it became symbolic of a juvenile 'crime wave'. Because the murder occurred outside the family it was taken as the strongest evidence of a breakdown in traditional moral values. The 'folk devils', the young murderers, were reported as 'other', and portrayed as symptomatic of a dislocated and collapsing society. They represented the sharp end of a continuum of violence endemic in childhood/ youth culture.

While adult child killers and abusers, together with their victims, were pathologized and located beyond 'normal relations', the James Bulger murder was a 'street crime'. In this case all children were at risk. The ubiquitous threat attached to representations of juvenile street crime was combined with the horrific extremity of child killings usually confined to the private domain. Further, not only were all children in any social setting vulnerable, there were no accurate indicators of the potential sources of danger. Because the killers were children, the conceptualization of 'stranger danger' was undermined. As Hay explains;

Our inability to distinguish between the face of the 'juvenile delinquent' and that of 'innocent youth' stimulates a profound sense of
anxiety and insecurity as conventional conceptions of innocence and
guilt become deeply problematised (1995:198).

Prior to the arrest and conviction of the two boys, many Merseyside
parents were not only confronted with the possibility that their child could be
at risk, but that he could have been one of the killers. It was an anxiety that
lived on after the convictions:

We will never be able to look at our children in the same way
again . . . All over the country, parents are viewing their sons in a new
and disturbing light. Where we see them at the ages of 9, 10 or 11,
pushing each other, jostling, or showing impatience with their
younger brothers and sister, we can't help wondering in what circumstances they could end up like . . . the killers of little James
Bulger . . . Parents everywhere are asking themselves . . . if the Mark
of the Beast might not also be imprinted on their offspring (*The
Sunday Times*, 28 November 1993).

Vulnerability and threat together resided in families. It is difficult to conceive
a story more powerful in its personal 'resonance', to use Hay's (1995) term. It
is also difficult to conceptualize media coverage in which children asked themselves if the adults close to them might be 'imprinted' with the 'Mark of the
Beast'.

Also significant in the story's power and its coverage was its visibility. The
abduction was caught on camera, the pictures frozen and enhanced. It was
witnessed by more than 30 adults who remembered seeing James Bulger being
led to his death. Yet the visibility of the crime showed the abductors to be
ordinary, indistinguishable from other children. It was a consistent theme
before and during the trial. Yet there was an expectation, almost a desire, for
those responsible to look different from ordinary or 'normal' boys (*Daily
Express*, 25 November 1993). The murder of James Bulger, particularly the
visibility of the crime and the 'ordinariness' of the perpetrators, created a
powerful sense of anxiety. The panic was fuelled and the story was transformed from a specific, aberrant murder to a symbol of national malaise and
social breakdown. Yet the crime, a child killed by another child/children, was
rare. Ironically, the regularity of the murder of children by adults was overshadowed by one unusual, tragic murder. The 'crisis', rather than being one of
adulthood became one of childhood.

Following initial reporting of the abduction and murder of James Bulger
and the search for those responsible, the media turned its focus on the 'deepening crisis' concerning young people and lawlessness. The case soon became
a metaphor for a structural, creeping malaise infecting the roots of British
society. From February 1993 through to November, when the two boys were

convicted of murder, the James Bulger case remained a significant news story. Once the boys had been named and their photographs published, the key theme of pathological 'evil', a reference made by the trial judge, was pursued relentlessly. For the *Daily Mirror* (25 November 1993), the two boys were 'Freaks of Nature', and given 14 pages of coverage. Though the photographs showed 'the faces of normal boys . . . they had hearts of unparalleled evil.' The *Daily Star* (25 November 1993) followed its front page question, 'How Do You Feel Now You Little Bastards?' with nine pages of coverage. The *Sun* (25 November 1993) echoed the theme of evil. Its front page headline proclaimed that the 'Devil Himself Couldn't Have Made A Better Job Of Two Fiends' and ran the story over 15 pages.

The media had difficulty in reconciling the horror of the crime and its circumstances with the ordinariness of the two boys. For example, a *Daily Express* (25 November 1993) reporter stated:

> From my seat at the front of Crown Court number one, I was one of the few reporters . . . who could see the faces of the two schoolboys accused of killing James. They were not what I expected . . . It was difficult to reconcile their innocent looks with the nightmare of James's death . . .

While 'evil' was the theme underpinning explanations for the murder, it was subsumed by a search for the 'cause' of a broader 'crisis' in childhood. Throughout the period between the murder and the trial the theme of 'crisis' prevailed yet the media had no specific subjects to analyse. Thus the 'evil' of children, undisciplined and out of control, contextualized the trial. In this scenario there was no consideration of the realities and experiences of the young boys or of their childhoods. Janet Daley (*The Times*, 25 November 1993) illustrates the point:

> what happened to him [James Bulger] seems to me not an incomprehensible freakish incident but simply the worst possible example of amoral childish viciousness; horrible precisely to the degree that it was childlike – random, aimless and without conscience . . . If we are all 'guilty', it is of refusing to accept the naturalness of evil and that all adults – even the reluctant and cowardly – must be held responsible for keeping it in check.

Walter Ellis (*The Sunday Times*, 28 November 1993) was typical in his apocalyptic references to Golding's *Lord of the Flies* (see also leader comment, *Daily Mail*, 25 November 1993; *Independent*, 25 November 1993):

> The widely held theory . . . is that evil is not innate but that nurture, temptation and the ills of society call it into being . . . I think, after the Bulger case that I no longer believe this.

Yet Ellis conflated this biological determinism with a behavioural determinism:

> The unique feature of the Bulger case remains its wanton desecration of innocence. Parents must certainly learn to discipline their children. Schools must restore at least some neglected values.

What was invidious about this line of argument was the portrayal of childhood evil as the enemy within the child. The invisible sign or mark had to be revealed, as if engaged in a mediaeval witch-hunt. Ellis continued:

> The trouble is, as we look at children playing, with a frisson of apprehension and fear that was not there before, that we can never know which of them has the Satan Bug inside him (sic) . . . They all look the same. But somehow they all look different.

In this portrayal, *all* children are suspect, potentially biologically infected. As Ros Coward (*Observer*, 28 March 1993) argues, such diatribes were underpinned by deeply-held yet simplistic stereotypes of childhood: 'When adults insist that a "proper" child is an angel with no sexuality, no aggression, no cruelty, then constitutional "evil" becomes the only way of understanding lies, destructiveness and cruelty.'

In support of the claim that childhood was in crisis the media used statistics, anecdotal evidence, appeals to common-sense and, as ever, 'experts'. Yet there was no agreement even over the juvenile crime statistics (*Guardian*, 18 February 1993). While police statistics showed an increase in juvenile crime of 54 per cent, the Home Office showed a fall in the juvenile crime rate. In fact statistical evidence in support of a deepening crisis was notable by its absence. Frances Crook (*Guardian*, 18 February 1993), of the Howard League, offered one of the few dissenting views to the pre-eminent theme of a nation overwhelmed by juvenile crime. She claimed that politicians were confusing serious crimes with persistent offending, that murders by young people were 'too small to generalise'. She also argued that incidents in which children were killed by strangers were rare:

> It is hardly credible that discussion about the moral malaise in the country should have focused on one case of a killing, however dreadful. The profound economic and social problems we face deserve a higher level of discussion. The people who are always condemned are inner-city children from poor families. Children of 12 and 13 are being made into scapegoats, even an enemy within (*Guardian*, 18 February 1993).

Similarly, Nick Cohen (*Independent on Sunday*, 21 February 1993) noted that since 1982 on average just one under-five child per year had been killed by a stranger. Of the 70-plus children murdered each year, most were killed by parents or adults known to them (*Independent on Sunday*, 21 February 1993). Even when there was some balance to the statistical analysis, some journalists sought reinforcement for their pet theories. Melanie Phillips (*Observer*, 28 November 1993) quoted the 'experienced voice' of Professor Elizabeth Newsom, head of the Child Development Research Unit at Nottingham University, who warned, 'The figures are very small now, but what frightens me is that we may be on the verge of something much bigger.'

The evidence, that serious crimes committed by children were aberrations, cut no ice as well-established journalists persisted with their construction of a 'national malaise'. Distinct and unrelated events were conflated to construct a notion of general crisis which, in turn, was further elaborated by politicians and 'experts'. Using logos and banner headlines, the tabloid press pulled together quite different stories of young people, many of which would not have been reported nationally in more usual circumstances. In the *Daily Express* (24 February 1993) Gordon Greig claimed that the Government was ready to answer the 'wave of public horror over spiralling crime'. The *Daily Express* suggested a spectre of 'Britain in Fear', filling its front page with the headline '54 crimes in fifty days – Police can't stop a city's young thugs'. It was alleged that children had committed these crimes while held at a children's home in Nottingham. The inside pages of the same edition presented a new logo, 'Violent Britain', and produced a 'snap survey' of juvenile crime in Britain. The coverage announced the 'impotency of current laws' in dealing with 'persistent joyriders, car thieves, shoplifters and tearaways who prey on young children and the elderly'. The survey proclaimed more 'horrifying examples of juvenile crime' (*Daily Express*, 24 February 1993). At Liverpool's juvenile court, for example, 'boys as young as ten faced a range of charges including stealing cars, assault and burglary.' It reported seven Hampshire teenagers questioned by the police for beating up another youth. In Worthing a boy of 13 was one of a gang of young people accused of burglary and joyriding. In the West Midlands 'violence, truancy and alcohol consumption are rife among teenagers on council estates.' In Sheffield 'children as young as twelve are being sent out on shoplifting sprees by older criminals.' The newspaper made no attempt to draw distinctions between these cases but used them as a collective demonstration of its argument that the national malaise of lawlessness among Britain's youth had consolidated.

The leader in the *Daily Telegraph* (22 February 1993), citing the Bulger case, reflected the common theme:

A mental state of pessimistic fatalism has the country in its grip. The sense of national despondency is not purely political and economic . . . but spans almost the entire range of human experience . . . The sense that things have rarely been as bad and can only get worse is now a major influence holding back recovery from recession . . . The existence of a bedrock of decency means the foundations are still there to be built upon. It is to this moral reconstruction that attention must now turn.

Highly subjective anecdotal accounts were used to confirm the crisis. An article, by novelist Beryl Bainbridge (*Daily Mail*, 20 February 1993), described her return to Liverpool. She witnessed young children whose

> countenance was so devoid of innocence that I was frightened. They were old beyond their years and undeniably corrupt. Women passing by said – there's more of them than there used to be, they should have been drowned at birth.

The following day the Prime Minister added his voice to the concern.

> 'I would like the public to have a crusade against crime and change from being forgiving of crime to being considerate to the victim. Society needs to condemn a little more and understand a little less' (*Mail On Sunday*, 21 February 1993).

From the abduction and murder of a young child a 'crisis' of national significance, reported internationally, was constructed. Lynda Lee Potter was unequivocal in her assessment of the problem:

> we seem to be speeding ever faster to a nightmarish world where children rarely go to school, roam the streets 'til midnight, know how to roll a joint, gloat over sick videos and think fun is tying a firework to the tail of a cat and setting it alight . . . We have a world where children are growing up virtually as savages (*Daily Mail*, 26 November 1995).

The sheer volume of media reporting, asserting public horror and helplessness in the face of 'the rise in crime' and the perceived increasing 'nastiness' of young people, led the media to search for the 'cause' of the decline. Richard Lynn, Professor of Psychology (*Daily Mail*, 22 February 1993), identified the decline as reflecting a 'helpless society, helpless to confront the crime which makes our lives a misery in so many parts of the country, helpless to maintain standards of decency, helpless to reverse the trend.'

This helplessness was identified as being part of an institutional malaise in which the state had gone 'soft' on criminals and offenders, neglecting discipline and punishment. The spectre of 'persistent young offenders' caused the Home Secretary, Kenneth Clarke, to state that the Government had failed to tackle the 'root of the crisis'. He suggested that:

> the courts should have the power to send really persistent nasty little juveniles away to somewhere where they will be looked after

better . . . John Major and I believe it is no good that some sections of society are permanently finding excuses for the behaviour of the section of the population who are essentially nasty pieces of work (*Daily Mail*, 22 February 1993).

Lynn considered that the decline in discipline was family-related:

The old fashioned wisdom about the importance of a stable loving and disciplined home background turns out to have sound scientific basis . . . My view is that the growth of crime in this country is because the concept of punishment has been all but abolished. It is unfashionable, it raises liberal hackles, and yet there are scientific reasons to believe that discipline and punishment can modify behaviour (*Daily Mail*, 22 February 1993).

The Archbishop of Canterbury Dr George Carey (*Daily Express*, 23 February 1993) suggested that the murder of James Bulger had 'brought to the surface the growing worries of so many who fear that there is a moral malaise at the heart of our society . . . crime levels are soaring.' Lack of discipline and assumed but vague decline in 'family values' were linked to the physical breakdown of the nuclear family and growth in one-parent families. Melanie Phillips called for a return to family values, arguing that children brought up by one parent were at greater risk as two parents were needed to deal with the 'collapse of moral certainty'. She argued the superiority of the two-parent family in disciplining children, claiming that a 'father is a vital necessity for a child's emotional health' (*Observer*, 13 June 1993).

Similarly, Charles Murray (1993), American sociologist and guru of the Right, argued for the 'link between lone parenthood and specific social problems' and that research would establish 'that after all children of lone parents are more criminal than children from two-parent families.' For Murray, the father taught 'his son crucial lessons about restraint and responsibility':

In neighbourhoods with lots of fathers those groups [to which young males want to be a part] tend to be clubs with adult male leadership, whereas in neighbourhoods filled with single mothers, those groups tend to be gangs with the morality that Golding described in *Lord of the Flies*.

It seems that the presence of lone mothers would not have made much difference on Golding's Pacific isle. Murray's solution was the abolition of welfare and child support, thus reviving 'social stigma' against single parents.

Having established that young people were incapable of distinguishing between right and wrong, the 'experts' then targeted the 'failing' education system. Contemporary education had become side-tracked by offering choice and emphasizing imagination. According to Philosophy Professor, Anthony

O'Hear, (*Daily Mail*, 19 March 1993), education encouraged children to, 'make choices and express views' before they were ready and capable. The priority, before choice and expression, should be 'virtuous conduct'. The cause of the assumed decline in education standards, as with the family, was placed firmly at the door of leftist progressives who had encouraged a decline in 'moral education'. The opinions of repentant 'ex-progressives' were used to support this argument. 'Reformed socialist', Professor A. H. Halsey, argued that the Labour Party was responsible for 'decades of failure on schooling and moral values.' Ignoring the impact of successive Conservative governments, Halsey considered that 'teachers, like parents – were now reluctant to take as much responsibility for pupils' moral education as they should' (*Daily Mail*, 24 February 1993).

The Education Secretary, John Patten, warned of the 'battle ahead to bring youngsters under control' adding that 'we face a very long haul of five to ten years before we undo some of the changes of the sixties and seventies' (*Daily Express*, 23 February 1993). Truanting was added to the debate, following evidence that the boys convicted of murdering James Bulger were absent from school. Patten equated truancy with crime: 'Show me a persistent truant and we have someone at risk of becoming a criminal' (*Daily Express*, 23 February 1993). He drew support from the *Daily Telegraph* (23 February 1993), which reported that the 'vast majority' of youth crime was committed by children between 14 and 16 'absconding' from school. Truancy was an issue which spanned the political divide between newspapers. In the *Guardian* (18 February 1994) Joanna Coles voiced her concern over children's 'vulnerability'. She contested Liberty's (Formerly National Council for Civil Liberties) criticisms of police involvement with anti-truancy schemes:

> kids have another right of which . . . [Liberty] . . . should be reminded. They have the right to be protected from older kids and adults who mean them harm . . . No matter how tough they feel inhaling Camels down the arcade, children have no sense of how vulnerable they really are.

Coles ignored contextual issues such as the non-criminal nature of truancy, the value of schooling or schools as 'safe' places, concluding that if children 'do not come to school of their own accord, we must go out and fetch them.'

In its search for 'causes' of childhood deviance in general and, after their trial, the motivations of the boys who killed James Bulger in particular, the media gave prominence to 'video nasties'. The Secretary of State for Wales had raised this issue soon after the murder (*Mail on Sunday*, 28 February 1993), noting:

> a generation bombarded by TV images of gratuitous violence, loveless sex and amoral behaviour – or hooked on computer games. Where a previous generation looked up to Bobby Moore, today's young people are more concerned with synthetic flickering video

images. The average teenager today has seen something like 30,000 killings on the cinema and TV screen . . . If that doesn't lead to delinquency, what does?

Lorraine Fraser, medical correspondent of the *Mail on Sunday*, claimed that research by the Royal College of Psychiatrists had established a link between video/TV violence and child murders and sex offenders. She concluded, 'There is good evidence now that susceptible children are affected by video violence and pornography. Hundreds of thousands of children have already been affected' (*Mail on Sunday*, 28 February 1993). This research found that 25 per cent of adolescent murderers and violent sexual offenders had repeatedly watched 'violent or pornographic' videos before committing their crimes. Dr Susan Bailey (quoted in *Mail on Sunday*, 28 February 1993), who conducted the research, identified the problem as lack of control:

The young adolescent murderers I have seen were out of control in the home, the community and education. Part of that being out of control may have involved access to these videos. That forms part of the critical pathway to what they do.

Despite the certainty of her concluding comment, Dr Bailey's tenuous connection that children 'may' have had access to videos hardly constituted a reliable finding. Further, two important questions were not asked. If videos were thought to be harmful, why was this harm restricted to children? And why were video images of violence thought to be so damaging when the infliction of *real* violence on children was ignored? Such acts of violence were not referred to as violence, but as 'discipline' or 'punishment', a distinction not considered worthy of mention, let al.one analytical attention.

The threat of societal breakdown was also considered by James Ferman, Director of the British Board of Film Classification (*Mail on Sunday*, 28 March 1993). Citing the Bulger case and calling for more legislation to 'help parents look after their children', he argued:

Only if parents are properly informed can they supervise what their children view. It is vital that parents take responsibility for what their children watch. If we don't look after our children – the most vulnerable element in society – we could go the way of American cities . . . if this threat to our children is not tackled soon, it may be too late.

The hysteria over video nasties was brought to a head at the trial's conclusion. The judge, Mr Justice Moreland, in ruling that the boys should be detained for 'very many years', declared, 'It isn't for me to pass judgement on their upbringing but I suspect that exposure to violent films may in part be an explanation' (*Daily Mirror*, 25 November 1993). The trigger for this renewed worry was the fact that videos, including *Childs Play 3* had been found at the home of one of the boys. David Alton, a Merseyside Liberal MP, demanded a Home Office investigation into the role played in the case by TV and video violence (*Daily Mirror*, 25 November 1993). He claimed that one of the boys had access at home to over 400 videos, 64 of which contained violence or soft pornographic material. For Alton, 'It is crucial that the nation searches its soul and asks how this kind of crime can happen and what are the causes of this unspeakable violence in our society' (*Daily Mirror*, 25 November 1993).

While asserting the 'causes' of the 'crisis' in childhood, the media also offered suggestions for its solution. Not surprisingly, these reflected the over-whelmingly reactionary framework within which the 'crisis' had been identi-fied and explained. From calls for a return to National Service (*Daily Telegraph*, 22 February 1993) to Melanie Phillips' 'caring' response based on family regimes of 'Tough Love' (*Observer*, 13 June 1993), solutions were predicated on the assumptions that society was collapsing into lawlessness due to a 'decline' in moral values. They were responses grounded in the orthodoxy of adult dominance. Politicians of all parties competed within this climate of reactionary fervour. Tony Blair, then Shadow Home Secretary, called for a national campaign to deal with the 'crisis' and for the expansion of secure accommodation for young offenders (*Daily Telegraph*, 22 February 1993). The Home Secretary, Kenneth Clarke, offered a 'crime crackdown' to be spear-headed by private security firms brought in to run detention centres for the 'new generation of under-15 criminals' (*Liverpool Daily Post*, 23 February 1993). Conservative MP Ivan Lawrence, Chair of the All-Party Home Affairs Select Committee, argued that what was needed was a 'return to approved schools where they are punished, taught discipline and educated' (*Daily Telegraph*, 22 February 1993). In accord with this tide of reactionary opinion, ex-High Court Judge Sir Fredrick Lawton, demanded a return to corporal punishment to 'whip young thugs into line' (*Daily Star*, 23 February 1993). Clifford Longley (*Mail on Sunday*, 28 February 1993) asked, 'Does society any longer have the courage to impose discipline on youth, to punish infractions with the traditional mix of drill, hard labour and humiliation, thereby to make boys into men?' For Longley the problem lay in the neglect of the moral education of the young, for 'National Service is an idea whose time has still not yet completely gone.' The author Alan Sillitoe reflected the prevailing climate suggesting that young people should know the difference between right and wrong, concluding that 'the only way to stop young criminals is to lock them up, for our good as well as theirs' (*Daily Mail*, 15 March 1993). In the wake of this reaction Suzanne Moore *(Guardian*, 26 March 1993) concluded that chil-dren 'have only to look around them to see that ours is a culture that does not actually like children very much.'

Two years after the conviction of the two boys, political concern with the supposed undermining of 'family values' remained a central issue within the media (see 'Who Killed the Family?', *BBC2*, 31 October 1995). Yet the media failure to address the key issue of violence *within* the idealized traditional family was thrown into sharp relief by media reaction to the report of the independent Commission on Children and Violence set up by the Gulbenkian Foundation after James Bulger's murder. In contrast to the dominant media and political comment surrounding the case, its findings focused on the role of physical 'punishment' in families and its relationship to later violent behaviour. Predictably, the media response was one of outrage. 'Fury at Call to Ban Smacking' was one front page headline (*Daily Express*, 10 November 1995). In its leading article the newspaper returned to 'leading psychologist' Professor Richard Lynn, who opined that:

> The objective of the commission is to abolish the last sanction on badly behaved children – the right of parents to administer physical punishment . . . If the commission succeed, the result will be a further breakdown of law and order and yet more crime.

The *Daily Mail* (10 November 1995) was also hostile to proposals to curb physical violence inflicted on children. Under the headline 'Report that's a Smack in the Face for Common Sense', Anthony Doran and Greg Hadfield wrote:

> Childcare specialist Lynette Burrows who believes the report should be consigned to the dustbin, accused the 'so-called progressive' authors of having crackpot views which had helped increase violence in society over the last ten years.

Former Chief Rabbi, Lord Jakobovits (*Daily Mail*, 10 November 1995), argued that parental violence represented an act of love. He stated, 'I smacked my children because I love them.' Reacting to the proposal for a charter of children's rights, he concluded:

> How sad! There has been far too much talk in our society of rights – what about duties? Why no charter of what children owe to their parents, as the Ten Commandments had it?

The *Sun* (10 November 1995) justified its support for familial violence by returning to the well-worn theme of child-centred anarchy:

> what has happened since the cane was abolished in schools?

> Teachers cower in front of pupils and parents are afraid to put their foot down for fear of offending their precious little darlings.

> Prisoners now insist that jails cannot be run without their full cooperation and delinquent youths are sent on safari. Society has gone soft and we are paying the price.

A gentle smack teaches a child there are punishments for those who break the rules.

Listen to the do-gooders and children will just run wild.

Conclusion

The outpouring of outrage and hatred against the boys convicted of James Bulger's murder had concrete effects on their case. First, there is little doubt that the trial jury would have been influenced by the extent, nature and tone of the media coverage between the murder date and the trial. Second, there is evidence that the press directly influenced the eventual sentence. *The Sun*, believing that the Judge's minimum recommended sentence of ten years was too short, began a campaign to have it increased. It asked readers to submit its published special coupons which stated that the boys should be imprisoned for longer. These were submitted to the Home Secretary. Subsequently he increased the term to a minimum of 15 years. According to a *Panorama* programme (*BBC1*, 9 October 1995), letters from the Prison Service stated that, 'In making his decision, the Secretary of State had regard to . . . the public concern about this case which was evidenced by the petitions and other correspondence.' When further pressed the Prison Service revealed that the 21,281 returned *Sun* coupons had been used as evidence of public concern. Trial, it seemed, was not directly by media, but the eventual sentencing was.

It is clear that double standards operate in the media portrayals of crimes committed by children and those committed by adults. Adults frequently kill young children, but media reactions are rarely of the seismic order of those following the killing of James Bulger. While such crimes as the latter are rare, the media has a ready template for their coverage. As shown in the discussion of St Saviours, this incorporates outrage, fears for social collapse, scapegoats for decline, appropriate 'expert' opinion, and even the same work of fiction, *Lord of the Flies*, referred to time and again as a verification of the fantasies of leader writers and columnists.

Quite different frameworks, however, are used for the reporting and discussion of the more widespread abuse and murder of children by adults. In this framework the wider implications are limited to local social services agencies, where social workers, characterized alternately as 'wimps' or 'bullies', are held publicly responsible for crimes they did not commit. Rarely is routine violence against children questioned. Indeed, it is encouraged within families as an instrument of 'discipline' and 'punishment'. The plight of families cast adrift into poverty as support services are cut is barely mentioned. Further, the masculinity of sexual abusers is conveniently ignored. Routine assaults on children are seen as the acceptable level of socializing and encouraging 'good' moral values. Occasionally violent crimes against children capture the headlines as some adults go 'too far' in exploiting the power relation that is theirs as an assumed right. But these are seen as excesses, as aberrations in a society which loves its children so much that they are legitimately and routinely assaulted.

Chapter 3

'Families' in 'Crisis'?

Vicki Coppock

The word *family* has enormous symbolic significance in contemporary British society. It evokes images which are uncompromisingly positive. The family represents all that is good and wholesome – the cornerstone of social life, 'a haven in a heartless world'. Society's health and well-being is assumed to be linked inextricably to that of the family. Yet, as the previous chapter demonstrates, the media carries the persistent message that 'childhood' is in 'crisis' and at the eye of the storm is the family. From across the political divide this message reverberates. According to Health Minister Peter Lilley, Britain is experiencing 'widespread collapse of the traditional family'. For Tony Blair, Leader of the Labour Party, it is a 'cycle of family disintegration, truancy, drug abuse and crime' (in Utting, 1995:6).

Demographic surveys indicate that since the early 1960s the popularity of marriage has declined significantly, with marriage rates at their lowest level since records began (OPCS, 1990, 1994a). Divorce rates for 1993 were at a new peak of 13.7 per thousand of the population, a sixfold increase since 1961 (OPCS, 1994a). Yet there has been an increase in cohabitation, with the number of first-married couples cohabiting prior to marriage rising from 6 per cent to 60 per cent over 25 years (Kiernan and Estaugh, 1993). Thirty-one per cent of births occur outside marriage, compared with 6 per cent in the early 1960s (OPCS, 1994b). In 1992 one in five families with dependent children were headed by a lone parent, compared to one in twelve in 1971 (OPCS, 1994b). The proportion of families headed by single women who have never married increased from 1 per cent to 7 per cent over the same period (Burghes, 1994; Haskey, 1994). In 1992, 67 per cent of mothers with dependent children were employed or seeking work, compared with less than 50 per cent in 1971. The greatest increase has been in mothers with preschool children with those 'actively' seeking paid work doubling to 50 per cent by 1992 (OPCS, 1994b).

Although many of these demographic trends in family living have emerged and consolidated over time, the public furore and sense of crisis is relatively recent (Jones, Tepperman and Wilson, 1995; Utting, 1995). Some commentators argue that the changes are a *cause* of social dislocation rather than a *symptom* (Davies, 1993; Dennis, 1993; Dennis and Erdos, 1992; Morgan, 1995; Murray, 1990, 1994). Feminism, inevitably, has been charged with vilifying the role of fathers (Morgan, 1986, 1995; Quest, 1992, 1994).

Others consider that families have become the *victims* of increasing individualism and materialism which has undermined the positive values of community and family (Coote, Harman and Hewitt, 1990; Hewitt and Leach, 1993). What these perspectives share, however, is an assumption that changes in the demographic make-up of families are, by definition, negative, pathological and detrimental to society as a whole.

As shown in Chapter 1, critical analyses have challenged such traditional common sense assumptions, revealing the family to be an historical and cultural creation (Anderson, 1983, 1995; Donzelot, 1980; Gittins, 1985). As an ideological construct, the 'family' has become enshrined in state policies, the law and professional practices (Barrett and McIntosh, 1982; Smart, 1984, 1989). Consequently, the family became established as the cornerstone of 'national childhood', underpinning the crucial structural relationship between the 'private' and 'public' domains. This chapter critically examines the traditional nuclear family as the primary context for child-rearing, revealing how its idealization masks the significance of power relations based on age, class, ethnicity and gender. An exploration of the boundaries between the state (public) and the family (private) illustrates how it remains central to contemporary British social policy and legislation, defining and regulating relationships and responsibilities. Contemporary discourses which proclaim that children's rights within the family have been secured are scrutinized, their contradictions and tensions revealed in the light of the lived experiences of children and young people.

The Traditional Family in Context

Anthropologists and sociologists have established that the family has always existed in some form and variations can be found in all societies. However, 'because the family seems to be the predominant unit we must not be bemused into thinking that it is the "natural" or "basic" one' (Fox in Edholm, 1991:141). Critical anthropological research has indicated that the family is only one specific form in the organization of reproductive and socializing relationships between parents and children, and between men and women. As Edholm states:

> Universal definitions of human relations must be constantly questioned and the whole notion of 'natural' must, in terms of human relations, be challenged, and the 'unnatural' – in these terms the social construction of relationships – must be fully recognized (1991:141).

For more than 150 years the ideal of the middle-class Victorian family has dominated British social life. The emergence of the modern family as a concept and as an ideological construct has been traced to the development of the industrial bourgeoisie during the later stages of capitalist development (Lewis, 1986). In contrast to the feudal, pre-industrial extended family where several generations were assumed to co-reside, being materially dependent on each other, the modern industrial nuclear family is a significant departure, being conjugal, private and self-centred (Parsons, 1949, 1955).

In early capitalism, the growing affluence of the bourgeoisie and its decreasing need for family labour in the production process necessitated the adaptation and modification of scientific and religious notions of masculinity, femininity, adulthood and childhood. The husband/father became the 'natural' head of the household, with wife and children as both economic and political dependants. Thus, 'by the end of the nineteenth century hearth and home had become the chief prop of a moral order no longer buttressed by religious belief' (Lewis 1986:31). Victorian philanthropists sought to reform and 'save' the working classes through a system of moral teaching which emphasized family life, maternal care, domesticity and privacy (Pearson, 1975; Stedman Jones, 1977; Woodroofe, 1962).

As the middle classes gained political influence, so family ideology was enshrined further in state policies and legal processes (Donzelot, 1980; O'Donovan, 1985; Rose, 1987; Smart, 1984). Laws on marriage, the ownership of property, child custody and taxation are each examples of the institutionalization and reproduction of particular family structures, consolidated throughout the twentieth century (Smart, 1991). The bourgeois family has permeated virtually every social institution in the interests of securing stability in the public sphere as well as the private (Dallos and McLaughlin, 1993; Frost and Stein, 1992). The structural functionalist analyses of Bronislaw Malinowski (1927), Kingsley Davis (1948), George Murdock (1949) and Talcott Parsons (1949, 1955) dominated post-war analysis of the family. Their main assumptions included: *universality*, that the family fulfils the functional prerequisites for the survival of human societies (reproduction, maintenance, social placement and socialization of the young); *naturalness*, that the family is biologically given; the division of gender into a language of *instrumental* (man as the provider of material resources) and *expressive* (woman as the provider of emotionality and caring) roles; the family as a private refuge from the harsh realities of the public world of work (see also: Dennis, Henriques and Slaughter, 1956; Kerr, 1958; Young and Willmott, 1962). As Jane Lewis states:

> The bourgeois family with its bread-winning father and dependent wife, who performs the domestic labour for the household and cares for the young and old, is seen as an harmonious organic unit successfully meeting the needs of an industrial society (1986:32).

As outlined in Chapter 1, the ideology of the nuclear family was central to British social policy from the origins of the welfare state. It identified the family as the natural provider of care and support for its members (Land, 1976,

1978; Wilson, 1977). If men as breadwinners were economically active, then the needs and interests of women and children would be safeguarded. The Beveridge Report (1942) was clear that the state should provide social support and services in maintaining the family in its traditional form (Lewis, 1983; Zaretsky, 1976). Married women were insured through their husbands, their benefits dependent upon his employment record. Abel-Smith (in Wicks, 1991:173) notes the assumptions underpinning Beveridge:

- that marriages are for life: even if the parties do not stay together, the legal obligation to maintain persists until death or remarriage;
- that sexual activity and childbirth takes place, or at least should take place, only within marriage;
- that married women normally do no paid work or negligible paid work;
- that women and not men should do housework and rear children;
- that couples who live together with regular sexual relationships and shared expenses are always of the opposite sex.

In fact, the relationship of the family to the state was considered to be so natural and obvious that it attracted what Mishra (1984) calls a 'bipartisan political consensus'.

The extent of agreement within sociological theory about the family in this period also was significant, but should not be overstated. Debates took place concerning the nature of change between the pre- and post-industrial family and the extent to which the industrial nuclear family represented a 'march of progress' (Laslett, 1977; Laslett and Wall, 1972). Yet little attempt was made to develop a *critical* structural analysis of the family beyond that of its role and functions. Structural–functionalism contextualized the family, but *only* in these terms. Despite their differences of emphasis these conceptual frameworks each researched the family as though it was set apart from its wider social, political and economic contexts. Conflicts in relations within the family, and indeed between the various theoretical positions, were played down or ignored. This was not true of the more critical approaches which emerged in the late 1960s and early 1970s, most notably the feminist critiques.

An End to Consensus? Feminism and the Family

The feminist critiques, like those of feminism's first wave earlier in the century, challenged the role and function of the family and the sociological theories and research which prevailed. Within these critiques knowledge was identified as partisan, representing a male/patriarchal academic discourse which took for granted the politics of reproduction and its attendant gender roles (Smith, 1973). Contrary to positivistic assumptions, feminists refused to accept that research was 'a product of pure, uncontaminated factual awareness' (Stanley and Wise, 1983:154). Far from being neutral, traditional research into and knowledge about the family was identified as gender-biased, underpinned by *male* experiences and *male* definitions of knowledge and truth. The combination of epistemological crisis and the emerging women's movement paved the way for a new political consciousness and academic focus among women students, academics and researchers (Reinharz, 1993). New kinds of questions were asked and a new sociology of the family forged. The conceptualization of the family as a universal, biological inevitability gave way to an understanding of the family as an ideological and historical creation (Barrett, 1980; Lewis, 1986).

Just as they had been at the turn of the century, critical analyses of the family and efforts to change traditional family arrangements were central to the women's movement, both at the level of academic study and political action. Thorne (1982) identifies five themes central to a feminist rethinking on the family. *First*, feminists challenged prevailing assumptions, moving away from 'the monolithic model of the family' (Eichler, 1981:368) which assumes that emotional involvement, procreation, socialization and economic support occur legitimately and naturally only within a nuclear family setting. Rather, feminist research and writing revealed that such functions operate independently of each other, often outside of what is conventionally considered a family group. Moreover, there has been a celebration of the *diversity* of experiences which constitute family living, for example, same sex unions (Hanscombe and Forster, 1982; Hare, 1994; Levy 1992).

Second, feminists reclaimed the family as a subject for social and historical analysis, seeking to deconstruct the concept of family and focusing on underlying structures of sex and gender. Hartmann (1981), for example, has been highly critical of conventional family theory and research in so far as it defines the family as a unit possessing consistent and typical interests. In contrast, she argues that the family is a *location* for the production and redistribution of resources within which family members occupy unequal positions of power, therefore possessing conflicting interests. Delphy (1976), Hartmann (1981) and McIntosh (1981) have theorized how the unequal allocation of tasks within families are based on gender categories which favour men and capitalism and, therefore, form the basis of women's oppression (see also Barrett, 1980; Barrett and McIntosh, 1982; Ferri, 1993). Also significant have been those critiques of women's natural role within the family as childbearers and rearers, carers, and the defining of women by their reproductive status (see Ferguson, 1989; Finch, 1989; Finch and Groves, 1983; Finch and Mason, 1992; Firestone, 1972; Land, 1978; Oakley, 1979; O'Brien, 1981; Rich, 1977; Ungerson, 1989). While there has been considerable debate concerning analytical and political standpoints, leading to the development of 'feminisms', there is a consistent recognition of the significance, both in the private and public domains, of *patriarchy* as an overarching determining context of women's oppression, regulation and control (see Coward, 1983; Millett, 1970; Smart and Smart, 1978; Walby, 1990).

Third, feminists have explored the differentiation of family experiences previously mystified by family ideology, exposing the realities of conflict, violence and inequality. They have challenged the notion of 'family as safe haven' using primary research based on the experiences of women and children within families. Such research has demonstrated that the nature and extent of male physical and sexual violence against women and children in the family is wide-ranging, systematic and severe (see Brownmiller, 1976; Dobash and Dobash, 1980, 1992; Feminist Review Collective, 1988; Gelles and Cornell, 1990; Gordon, 1989; Kelly, 1988; Radford and Russell, 1992; Stanko, 1985).

Fourth, feminists have problematized the concepts of private and public social worlds. At one level, the separation of 'family' (private) and 'society' (public) is challenged as 'partly illusory, since there are close connections between the internal life of families and the organisation of the economy, the state, and other institutions' (Thorne, 1982:3). At another level, however, there has been a recognition of the negative consequences of this false separation for women and children, who are often isolated behind closed doors, cut off from outside contact and support (Dobash and Dobash, 1992; Edwards, 1989; Mama, 1989; Pahl, 1985).

Fifth, feminist analysis has opened up debate around the tensions between values of 'market-based individualism' and 'family-based nurturance' (Thorne, 1982:3). Within the liberal feminist tradition, women have historically fought for individualism and equality, although for some feminists these values are uncomfortably close to those of capitalism. Values of nurturance and collectivity have been celebrated as womanly and family-centred and held in direct opposition to man-made, worldly qualities of the public sphere (see Bridenthal, 1982; Gordon, 1982; Rich, 1977; Zaretsky, 1982).

The impact of feminist critiques of the family has been considerable. Not only did they question and deconstruct family life, but also demonstrated that the relationship between the state and the family is far from politically or ideologically neutral. Rather, this relationship has been revealed as value-laden, underpinned by familiar assumptions which have rarely been questioned in standard sociological theory (see David, 1986; Delphy and Leonard, 1992; Glendinning and Millar, 1987; Graham, 1984; Land, 1983; Land and Rose, 1985; Showstack-Sassoon, 1987; Wilson, 1977). Yet this contribution has not been welcomed universally. Since the changing political context of the late 1970s, 'feminist theories and thinking have mainly been in dialogue with anti-feminist or New Right theories and policies on the family' (David, 1993:15). While the basic ideological and political premises of the traditional nuclear family have permeated all political agendas this century, the 1979 election of the Conservative Party under the leadership of Margaret Thatcher marked a significant intensification of family ideology within British government and politics. Therefore, 'even where rhetoric is relatively unchanging, there is always a different political significance to such discourses which derives from the economic, political and social climate in which they gain ascendancy'

(Smart, 1991:153–4). A decisive and defined political and ideological agenda within Thatcherism impacted on the state–family relationship in contemporary Britain and is crucial to understanding the construction of 'the family in crisis' in the 1990s.

Which is the Party of the Family?

In the 1980s right-wing politicians and their academic advisers came to dominate debates concerning the family in Britain. The New Right consolidated its political influence, arguing that the welfare state had become too large, too expensive, too bureaucratic and ineffective. Concern was expressed with the permissiveness of the 1960s and 1970s and, as Chapter 2 shows, political debate centred on powerful notions of declining morality and family values (Mount, 1982; Scruton, 1986). Such sentiments underpinned the clandestine activities of Prime Minister Thatcher's Family Policy Group whose existence was only brought to public attention via a series of Cabinet papers leaked to the *Guardian* newspaper (*Guardian*, 17 February 1983). This group was responsible for secretly drafting a series of radical proposals for welfare policy reform aimed at strengthening the family (see Abbott and Wallace, 1992; Durham, 1991).

Demographic changes in family life (for example: increased divorce, co-habitation, lone parenthood, 'illegitimacy', working mothers) were identified as socially and morally wrong. They were attributed to the political aims (and assumed failure) of post-war liberal welfarism which had encouraged the destabilization of the traditional nuclear family by pandering to the political demands of civil rights and liberation movements. The 'normal' family had been undermined within a 'lobby-ridden society' (Anderson and Dawson, 1986:9). It was maintained that these changes have had profound consequences for the *economic* as well as the moral well-being of the nation. As stated earlier, they are represented as a cause rather than a symptom of social dislocation, as it is claimed that the decline of the traditional family has generated social ills including the emergence of a 'dependency culture', an 'underclass', rising crime, delinquency, homelessness, child abuse and neglect and HIV/AIDS (Dennis, 1993; Dennis and Erdos, 1992; Murray, 1990, 1994; Segalman and Marsland, 1989).

Much of the political rhetoric concerning the changes in families is derived from the influential ideas of a small group of North American and British commentators (from both the New Right and the 'Ethical Left') whose writings have been published and publicized by the Institute of Economic Affairs. A common theme is the call for a reduction in 'unnatural' state intervention because of its perceived adverse effects on the natural family and community. As Segalman and Marsland state:

> The welfare-dependent family in the urban ghetto . . . is unable to produce children adequately equipped to re-enter society and the

labour market without considerable difficulty and disturbance ...
the availability of welfare has itself contributed to welfare dependency and ghetto social pathology (1989:45).

The right-wing American social scientist Charles Murray (1984, 1989,
1994) argues that liberal welfare policies have encouraged dependency and
reduced levels of individual responsibility, especially parental responsibility
for children (David, 1993). Murray is concerned about the emergence of what
he terms an 'underclass' of poor families predisposed towards crime, idleness
and the siring of 'illegitimate' children, and living outside mainstream society's
norms and values. Of particular focus is the growing number of never-married
mothers who rely on state welfare for their support.

> The question facing Britain is the same, haunting question facing the
> United States: how contagious is the disease? ... The *central
> truth ... is our powerlessness to deal with an underclass once it
> exists ... We don't know how to make up for the lack of good parents*
> (Murray, 1990:24, 33, emphasis added).

It is suggested that the 'normal' family has fallen foul of the welfarist
concern over 'abnormal' or 'problem' families, with normal families under
threat while 'less desirable' families drain scarce resources (Smart, 1991).
Moreover, it is assumed that increasing dependency on the family will of itself
restore social order and stability. As Paul Johnson, a right-wing political
commentator, states, 'The more society can be policed by the family and less
by the state, the more likely it is that such a society will be both orderly and
liberal' (*Observer*, 10 October 1982).

Predictably, feminism comes under attack for poisoning women's attitudes towards men, marriage and the family (Morgan, 1986, 1995; Quest, 1992,
1994), while the welfare state is criticized for facilitating women's withdrawal
from their traditional role through income maintenance policies for lone
mothers, relaxed divorce laws and legally sanctioned abortion. Gilder argues
that 'man has been cuckolded by the compassionate state' and proposes that
the state must change its economic and social relationship with women in
families. He continues, 'The woman's place is the home, and she does best
when she can get the man there too, inducing him to submit most human
activity to the domestic values of civilisation' (cited in David, 1993:18).

Such arguments are no longer the exclusive preserve of the New Right.
The emergence of the self-styled 'Ethical Socialists' (Norman Dennis, George
Erdos, A. H. Halsey) signalled a bizarre confluence of political and intellectual
thought from the Left and the Right. These authors believe that the traditional
family has been 'sold out' by the Left and the 1960s generation of liberal
intellectuals. They insist that it is the task of socialists to uphold family and
community ties, agreeing with New Right thinkers that the breakdown of the

traditional family is the problem. The phenomenon of 'families without father-hood' (Dennis, 1993; Dennis and Erdos, 1992) is considered to threaten the physical safety, psychological well-being and educational performance of children and young people. Such living arrangements are also held responsible for what is claimed to be an unprecedented escalation of anti-social and criminal behaviour in children and young people:

> The change to which we direct particular attention is the progressive liberation of young men . . . from the expectation that adulthood involves life-long responsibility for the well-being of their wife, and 15 or 20 years of responsibility for the well-being of their children. The hypothesis [is] that young men who are invited to remain in a state of permanent puerility will predictably behave in an anti-social fashion . . . (Dennis and Erdos, 1992:xxi).

> Adolescent boys are particularly vulnerable to paternal disengagement and absence. Far from ushering in a pacific and carefree Eden of exclusively feminine nurture, the banishment of fathers would condemn young males to underachievement at school and a life of violent crime outside it (Anderson and Dawson, 1986:14).

The preoccupation with the assumed failure of lone parent households, headed by women, to socialize male children is significant. There is no assumption that female children living in the same environment also might fall prey to delinquency, violence and underachievement. Clearly what is identified as most important is the reproduction of patriarchy and *male* culture through *male* children (Phillips, 1993).

As well as the strong quasi-religious discourse which runs throughout this literature, sociobiological theory is used to emphasize to the reader the naturalness of the nuclear family. Segalman and Marsland for example, maintain that the traditional nuclear family 'provides the child with two distinct and countervailing dynamic nuclei for his developmental life. Each of them is equipped by biological, psychological, anatomical and hormonal qualities to perform the necessary services for the child' (1989:40). Similarly, the work of Malinowski is resurrected in order to justify and inflict social stigma upon those who would deviate from the moral norm:

> I know of no single instance in anthropological literature of a community where illegitimate children, that is children of unmarried girls, would enjoy the same social treatment and have the same social status as legitimate ones . . . in all human societies moral tradition and the law decree that the group consisting of a woman and her offspring is not a socially complete unit (cited in Morgan, 1995:vi).

Although a unity of perspective is implicit in these arguments, Durham (1991) and Rodger (1995) warn that it is naive to assume that the influence of the New Right or the Ethical Socialists' agenda dictates that government policy and legislation will move harmoniously in a unified direction. Fundamental contradictions, at different times since 1979, have surfaced in successive Conservative administrations and their apparent confusion about whether they were sponsoring or constraining individualism in family life (for example, the recent obsession with the back to basics theme set alongside proposals for the introduction of no-fault divorces). In this Rodger suggests that the Government has struggled to accommodate the gulf between 'real movements' and 'ideological movements' in family life:

> The 'real movement' in family life is anchored in the complex dis-organising processes of late modern economies where the pace of technological change has transformed normative frameworks and social relationships, and is shifting relentlessly towards greater levels of negotiation and creativity in family and sexual relationships . . . However a contrary ideological movement . . . rooted in the political organisations of both the right and 'ethical left' has emerged with the objective of establishing the case that the well-being of children in particular, and human beings in general, is best preserved within a two-parent family based on heterosexuality . . . (1995:17–18).

Similarly, the economic and moral arguments of the New Right are not wholly consistent (Tame, 1991). Economic libertarianism urges state minimalism and a free market economy with a strong emphasis on the fundamental freedom and rights of all individuals. Conversely, traditional authoritarian conservatism advocates a pervasive centralized state committed to the maintenance of law, order and nationhood. Traditional patterns of authority which emphasize obedience and subservience to traditional principles, Christian values and the conventional family are seen as providing the solid foundation for society (Abbott and Wallace, 1992).

The representation of the family is crucial in understanding how this apparent contradiction is maintained. For, while 'the liberal objectives of reducing public welfare provision implies a traditional role for women and the family; conservatives provide an ideology for justifying such outcomes from public policy' (King, 1987:25). Ultimately, such interests are reconciled under patriarchal capitalism where the traditional family occupies a central ideological role in accommodating its inherent contradictions, tensions and crises. It is a world view which is classist, sexist, homophobic and racist in its assumptions. It represents a narrowly defined construction of the family based on white, western, middle-class ideals and norms. Groups who depart from these ideals and norms are defined as deviant, dangerous, or unnatural or alien (Cannan, 1992; Parton, 1991). Moreover, such sentiments are evident in a range of policies and legislative measures introduced by successive Conservative Governments since 1979 – paradoxically – given the call for a hands off approach to the family (see David, 1986; Durham, 1991; Fox-Harding, 1996; Rodger, 1995; Van Every, 1991).

Significantly, there is minimal evidence of any alternative discourse from either of the two main opposition parties in Britain. In fact in terms of political rhetoric their stances on the family remain indistinguishable from that of the New Right. Murray's theories on the underclass are afforded as much credence and concern by the Left as the Right. For example:

> I have no doubt that the breakdown in law and order is intimately linked to the breakdown of a strong sense of community. And the break-up of community, in turn, is to a crucial degree consequent upon the breakdown of family life (Tony Blair MP in Utting, 1995:6).

> If present trends continue many British children face a risky childhood. The combined force of single motherhood, children being born out of wedlock, divorce, remarriage and the rest means that by the year 2000 only about half of children in Britain will experience a 'conventional' childhood . . . (Malcolm Wicks Liberal Democrat MP, *Guardian*, 5 July 1993).

Despite the doomsday predictions of social calamity, there is little empirical evidence of 'significant differences across family types on measures of the socio-emotional adjustment and well-being of children' (Rodger, 1995:20). Moreover, historical research has revealed that, contrary to most of the morally judgmental commentary on the subject of the family, the twentieth century has been more conforming and stable than any previously documented century (Anderson, 1995).

Such expressions of anxiety or moral panics over the family are not new. Lewis (1986:31) argues that they are 'episodic responses to perceptions of actual or incipient family failure during periods of military or economic crisis.' She refers to the Boer War and the period immediately after the Second World War, suggesting that the nature of the anxiety changes over time, reflecting the development of knowledge and professional expertise about families. In particular, she notes the significance of changing ideas concerning the nature of poverty, the role of women and the importance of the mother–child relationship. Consequently, current anxieties about the family require contextualization in the material and economic changes of late modern society; a response to the inevitable restructuring of advanced industrial capitalism.

The Eternal Triangle: Children, Parents and the State

The theorizing, research and political debate concerning the family and 'childhood' has focused on, and has been conducted exclusively by, adults. Children have been either invisible or incidental objects of the adult gaze (Leonard, 1990). The position of chidren within the family is assumed to be secure and positive as long as the family fits the traditional, nuclear model. This consensual image has been increasingly challenged by critical theorists, particularly from within feminism, who have demonstrated that the family is a well-established site of oppression for children and young people.

Smart explains that children form part of a nexus of power within family relations – whether loved, cherished, neglected or abused. She states, 'Both mothers and fathers can be said to have power over children, whether this is economic power, physical power or emotional power' (1989:3). The status of parenthood establishes potential power claims over children through the vehicle of family law. Historically, childhood dependency has been codified in law in the form of parental rights. Rather than possessing rights themselves, children's recourse to law has been couched in terms of *protection*. Margolin (1978) suggests that the paternalistic tradition of the nineteenth century child-saving movement has persisted throughout the twentieth century, with the state intervening on behalf of children 'in their best interests', as a 'better parent' or when their families have been deemed to have 'failed' them (Frost and Stein, 1989; Parton, 1991; VACSG, 1990).

Intervening in the private domain of the home has always been controversial and poses a conundrum for the liberal state in so far as it brings into sharp focus the tension between the rights claims of the three parties involved – parents, children and the state. The state has avoided this inherent contradiction through the construction of the normal or functional family and its converse, the 'abnormal' or 'dysfunctional' family (Parton, 1991). Within the former an equilibrium of interests is assumed obviating the need for recognition of the separate rights claims of individual family members. Thus the state has become established as the supporter of parental (paternal) authority, the legitimator of adult–child power relationships, except when the exercise of that authority is deemed to be 'unreasonable' or 'inadequate'. Then it is classified as 'dysfunctional'. The state is able to maintain its legitimacy regarding the sanctity of the private sphere, while at the same time retaining a protectionist role in relation to children, through relationships of tutelage (Donzelot, 1980). Within this process state agencies and professionals have emerged as 'experts' defining and, under statute, regulating relationships and responsibilities within the family, straddling the split between the public and private spheres (Foucault, 1977; Rose, 1985, 1990). This is the context in which professional ideologies emerge and consolidate, informing and maintaining 'regimes of truth' and promoting official discourse as the only discourse (see Chapters 1 and 2).

Not only are the concepts of 'reasonable' or 'good enough' parenting inherently problematic, in so far as they invoke notions of *relative* rather than *absolute* abuse of power and authority, but also they are underpinned by the core features of family ideology – white, western, patriarchal, middle-class norms and values – as the standard against which *all* parenting is to be judged.

Consequently the construction of the dysfunctional family – that is any family deviating from the ideal – effectively disguises the reality of adult power as a problem in *all* families. This idealization of the family means that negative experiences within families are understood and constructed as problems with individual families or individuals within families rather than as negative aspects of the institution itself (Frost and Stein, 1989). As discussed in Chapter 1, the pathological 'disease model' of child abuse and neglect within the family has persistently dominated state policy, legislation and intervention in the lives of children and young people throughout the twentieth century. Therefore, the routine ordinariness of adult (usually male) power and violence within the family is diminished by theoretical assumptions and professional practices which attribute causation to 'deviant', 'dangerous' or 'pathological' individuals and families. As Sarah Nelson (1982) suggests, the clues reside in 'normal' family values, rather than 'deviant' or 'aberrant' values. They are prevalent throughout the history of pervasive authoritarian and punitive attitudes towards children in British society (Newell, 1989).

Things are done *to* children or *for* children by their families or the state. Their objectification exposes the assumption of childhood passivity which is at the heart of accepted interpretations of the oppression of children and young people. In such interpretations there is no sense in which children are considered to be independent actors within their environments. Any sign of them becoming 'active' learners or 'do-ers' is identified and represented as potentially dangerous. This is well-illustrated in the following quotation from the notorious but influential right-wing 'Black Papers' on education:

> Children are not naturally good. They need firm tactful discipline from parents and teachers with clear standards. Too much freedom for children breeds selfishness, vandalism and personal unhappiness (Cox and Boyson, 1975:1).

This statement typifies the internal contradictions within protectionist discourses. Any resistance to adult control is delegitimized and pathologized. It is for this reason that Kitzinger (1990) is cynical about some of the highly publicized preventative approaches to child abuse which encourage children to assert control and 'Say No'. She suggests that such methods are inadequate in so far as they fail to problematize the concept of childhood, arguing that 'It is not just the abuse of power over children that is the problem, but the existence and maintenance of that power itself' (1990:179). As Hood-Williams states, a new agenda in the social analysis of childhood is needed 'which presumes the existence of antagonistic relations within families and which focuses our attention onto the differential distributions of power, work, violence and rewards' (1990:159).

The 1990s: A Decade of Children's Rights?

Although discourses of paternalism and protectionism have dominated children's rights debates throughout the twentieth century, there has been resistance from those advocating the need for the recognition and expansion of the legal and moral rights of children and young people (CRO, 1995a, 1995b; CRDU, 1994; Franklin, 1986; Freeman, 1983). The broader, international civil rights movements of the 1960s and 1970s provided the radical context within which the position of children and young people in the family and other social institutions was problematized (Adams *et al.*, 1972; Farson, 1974; Holt, 1974). Specific instances of 'radical action' included student demonstrations, sit-ins and school strikes. Yet, while the movement was significant in opening up a vigorous debate around children's rights and childhood, and, as Chapter 5 shows, there were important developments in alternative schooling and 'deschooling', its specific impact was relatively limited. Paternalistic, protectionist assumptions remained all-pervasive.

The growth and activity of a number of pressure groups in the field of child care in the 1980s (National Association for Young People in Care; National Council for One Parent Families; Justice for Children; Children's Legal Centre; Family Rights Group; Parents Against Injustice; Dads After Divorce; Families Need Fathers) set alongside a number of key events (the Gillick Case; the inquiries into the deaths of Tyra Henry, Kimberley Carlile and Jasmine Beckford; Cleveland) increasingly drew attention to and created the impetus for a fundamental legal review of the different and often competing interests of family members. It was in this context that the 1988 Children Bill emerged, given Royal Assent in 1989 as the Children Act. Much was made of the new legislation's commitment to the rights of children. However, Eekelaar and Dingwall (1990) suggest that none of the official documents which led up to the 1989 Act addressed children's rights, even though this was a key issue among academics, practitioners and lobbyists seeking reform. One way of gauging any government's commitment to the empowerment of children and young people is to evaluate the impact of its legislation on their lives.

The 1989 Children Act created a uniform welfare principle giving statutory effect to the principle that the child's welfare is paramount and his or her wishes and feelings should be ascertained and taken into account by the court. Children can apply for the court's permission to be made parties in private proceedings and can make an informed decision regarding consent to any medical or psychiatric examination, or other assessment. Children in local authority care have a right to be consulted about any decisions affecting them; may apply to have any contact order refused; may, in certain circumstances, apply after 72 hours for an Emergency Protection Order to be discharged and may invoke complaints procedures.

While these changes appeared to encourage a shift in power from adults to children, the rhetoric of empowerment in the Act was significantly tempered by the qualification that the child must be of 'sufficient age and understanding' (the maturity test) to benefit from the potential increase in personal autonomy. Although a court may concede the basic principle that a *mature* child has the right to make certain decisions, this can be modified by a ruling which overrides the child's decision, if the court considers that decision to be detrimental to the child's welfare. In other words, the child's capacity to make a decision depends on an *adult* third party's assessment of the legitimacy of that decision through the same paternalistic mechanism of applying the 'best interests' rule.

Clearly this means that considerable opportunities remain for the continued imposition of adult values on children. Indeed, an accumulation of evidence following the Act's introduction indicates that such concerns are justified (see Bates, 1994; Children's Legal Centre, 1995; Clark, 1994; Fennell, 1992; Freeman, 1993; Lawson, 1991; Masson, 1991). The assumption that children are not really capable of reaching rational decisions, nor of exercising political power, prevails. Moreover, the principle of the child's welfare as paramount only applies in child care legislation, affecting only a minority of children.

The Act's introduction of the notion of *parental responsibility*, as opposed to *parental rights*, also is meant to signify a welcome move away from the idea of children as the possessions of their parents. Additionally it broadens the legal concept of parenting, acknowledging the role of unmarried fathers, cohabitees, grandparents, foster carers, local authorities and significant others. It recognizes that biological parents are not necessarily the most significant people in bringing up children. In fact there is only one definition of *family* in the Act. This 'includes any person who has parental responsibility for the child and any other person with whom he has been living' (Children Act 1989 s17(10)).

While there appears to be latitude in the interpretation of the concepts of parenting and family, the subsequent implementation through policy documentation and professional guidance has failed to match its promise. 'Nonconventionality' remains an indicator of 'bad parenting' (Van Every, 1991) and 'non-traditional' family forms persist as 'second best' (Cosis-Brown, 1991). Although the welfare principle is supposed to be the court's paramount consideration, frequently it appears more concerned with the sexuality of mothers than with the child's interests (Beresford, 1994). The parenting skills of non-biological lesbian and gay parents are marginalized and unrecognized (Hare, 1994; Jolly and Sandland, 1994; Levy, 1992). Overall, there remains an unwillingness 'to explore alternative familial forms, and to question the conceptual boundaries of "the family"' (Beresford, 1994:643).

Despite the apparently progressive rhetoric, the central ideological tenets of the Children Act can be traced to New Right thinking on the family. The perceived undermining of parental authority via permissive state education and welfare policies and professionals is manifested in the principle of 'nonintervention'. It represents the New Right vision of the family free from state interference, coping on its own. The Act created a major new duty for local authorities:

- to safeguard and promote the welfare of children within their area who are in need; and
- so far as is consistent with that duty, to promote the upbringing of such children by their families, by providing a range and level of services appropriate to those children's needs.

Yet it emphasizes the *voluntary* nature of arrangements between local authorities and families in the provision of services, meaning that their fulfilment depends significantly on adequate political will and resourcing. While this duty appears to signal a more positive approach towards family support and prevention, in that the definition of a 'child in need' allows for a wide interpretation, its implementation is fundamentally undermined.

Hearn (1995) has reviewed the findings of the 1993 *Children Act Report* and concludes that although the Act establishes a powerful case for prevention, a weak, fragmented approach to the promotion of children's welfare prevails alongside the persistence of a reactive social policing role. This has been confirmed by Utting (1995) who identifies the gap between imaginative legislation and inadequate implementation. Indeed, the new activity of child protection, as opposed to child care, confirms the New Right project of residualizing the state's responsibility for children's well-being, while at the same time strengthening its commitment to targeting 'deviant' or 'dangerous' families (Frost and Stein, 1989; Parton, 1991). What persists is the failure to recognize that relationships of dominance, subordination and exploitation are present in *all* families, leaving unaddressed the important broader issues concerning children and young people's civil rights and physical integrity within the family (CRO, 1995a).

A commitment to the restoration of the traditional authority of parents over children is re-packaged in the form of 'parental responsibility' – the means by which parents can retrieve what previously they lost to the state. The extent to which this authority ever was challenged, let alone lost, is a matter of dispute. Further, the gender-neutral term *parental* is misleading. The Act has been accused of facilitating a process of patriarchal reconstruction in so far as the granting of parental responsibility to unmarried fathers reflects the wider political and ideological agendas about 'families without fatherhood' discussed earlier (Dennis, 1993; Dennis and Erdos, 1992). O'Hara (1991) argues that men's power over women is inseparably linked to their power over children. She suggests that the British Conservative Government, via the legal system, has sought to maintain men's control over children while paying lip-service to concepts of children's rights.

Similar scepticism has been expressed regarding the United Nations Convention on the Rights of the Child. Adopted in 1989, but not ratified by the UK

Government until 1991, the Convention contains more than 50 articles covering every aspect of children's lives. It is the first detailed set of minimum standards against which governments can test their attitudes and practices towards children and young people. While essentially protectionist in its orientation, the symbolic significance and desirability of the Convention cannot be refuted. Its usefulness, however, can be judged only in terms of its impact on governments in practice. As with the 1989 Children Act, there is little evidence of positive UK Government action.

According to the Children's Rights Development Unit (CRDU, renamed in 1995 the Children's Rights Office), the non-governmental organization set up to monitor the implementation of the Convention in the UK, the British Government has failed to take seriously the Convention since ratification in 1991. Ironically, the British Government has contravened parts of the Convention, worsening the position of some children and young people through the introduction of repressive legislation (Criminal Justice Acts 1991, 1993; Education Act 1993; Criminal Justice and Public Order Act 1994). In January 1995 the UN Committee on The Rights of the Child met in Geneva to consider Britain's implementation of the Convention (UN Committee on the Rights of the Child 1995). It recorded its unequivocal and serious concern at the Government's failure to take children's rights seriously. In particular it criticized British law for permitting the 'reasonable chastisement' of children in the family, effectively sanctioning parental violence. Further, it expressed grave concern about the level of child poverty, homelessness and poor health in Britain.

Certainly, analysis of the British Government's approach to families since the late 1970s demonstrates a diminishing commitment to the general well-being of parents and children at the expense of an ideological and economic compulsion to cut public expenditure (Rodger, 1995). Utting emphasizes the heavy moralistic tone of the political rhetoric on internal family dynamics, as it diverts attention away from the wider structural influences on family life such as poverty and poor housing: 'The adverse consequences for children associated with that overall skewing of national wealth and prosperity away from families should be treated as a matter of profound concern' (1995:40). Research conducted by the Child Poverty Action Group (Middleton, Ashworth and Walker, 1994) supports this view, stressing the reality of childhood poverty in Britain in the 1990s and affirming the significance of class as a primary determining context in the lives of children and young people.

An Alternative Future for the Family?

As shown in the previous chapters and illustrated above, there has been a powerful wave of rhetoric concerning notions of 'childhood' and familial 'crisis' and this has dominated the focus of Government. It has served to divert attention away from a searching and critical analysis of the crucial issues, legitimating and strengthening the power and control of adults over children and young people. The rhetoric reflects and sustains a web of assumptions, both explicit and implicit, about the family, its constitution and its function. Family ideology, however, does not represent the reality of individuals living together. An ideology which claims that there is only one acceptable type of family cannot be matched in reality because it is no more than an 'ideal' not necessarily in tune with the ways in which people choose, or are able, to live their lives. It is the gap between ideology and reality which signifies the assumed 'crisis' in the family.

Those who subscribe to the 'breakdown of the family' thesis are concerned primarily with family *structures* and promoting a two-parent family 'ideal'. The narrowness of this perspective obscures an understanding of family *processes* and the qualitative (and quality) experiences of family members, particularly those of children and young people. Within the 'ideal' the social construction of compulsory heterosexuality as the only valid form of sexual relationship, expressed in the context of the nuclear family and underpinned by father-right, serves to legitimate and sustain relationships of power and dominance in the private sphere. Ultimately, any position which fails to acknowledge and address the existence of structural inequalities, both within and between families, in favour of some mythical notion of an unequivocally beneficial traditional nuclear family, remains fundamentally flawed.

Certainly there is potential within existing legislation for resistance and change. Those who work with children and families have for some time been aware that their notion of what constitutes a family has to widen, whether or not this fits with any particular ideological construction (Cosis-Brown, 1991). Rather than assuming that two parents must always be better than one, rather than scapegoating lone mothers and elevating the supposed contribution of fathers, there is a need to adopt a constructive interpretation of family living which focuses on parents and children as people, not problems (Utting, 1995). As Hanscombe and Forster conclude:

> Instead of spending millions on trying to find out what has gone wrong with the nuclear family, and how to rehabilitate it, we ought to spend these millions on finding out what domestic conditions will suit the people of the future better and how to achieve them (1982:158).

Chapter 4

Prolonging 'Childhood', Manufacturing 'Innocence' and Regulating Sexuality

Karen Corteen and Phil Scraton

No issue reveals the contradictions within the politics of childhood as starkly as that of sexuality, its definitions and regulation. As 'non-adults' children are assumed to be asexual. While they are socialized into gender-appropriate roles from birth, a universal feature of patriarchal societies, they are expected to retain a sexual naïvety. Yet the images which surround them, implicit and explicit, of hegemonic/dominant masculinity and emphasized/subordinate femininity are all-pervasive and all persuasive. The daily experiences of children and young people are contextualized by constructions of masculinity and femininity which are both gendered and sexualized. They are binary opposites whose binding attraction is generalized and homogenized on the basis of compulsory heterosexuality. The close association between the biology and politics of reproduction, albeit diverse in its specific cultural manifestations, normalizes and underwrites heterosexual relations. Just as gender implies relations of dominance and subordination, common throughout patriarchal societies, so heterosexuality reflects such relations. Historically, the material, social, cultural, political and physical oppression of women as gendered beings has been matched by the physical repression of women as sexualized beings. Any diversion from the social and cultural determining values has been interpreted and represented as a perversion. Beyond the context of 'servicing men', both economic and sexual, women's sexuality has no legitimacy – it is defined as abnormal or unnatural. As children develop they are expected to deal not only with their changing physicality and mixed emotions but also with the confused and confusing messages which govern their knowledge and understanding of the body, its 'normality' and its potential.

And the messages are confused. Television, newspapers, advertising, music and cinema guarantee a popular culture obsessed with heterosexual relations and intrigue in which the boundaries of fantasy and reality are purposefully blurred. Children and young people are expected to remain passive onlookers, locked within a kind of unquestioning childhood innocence. It is as if their age confers immunity from matters sexual, that by some mysterious process they will know the right time to ask appropriate questions and receive informed answers. Meanwhile, as adults-in-waiting they need protection. Protection from strangers, protection from evil, protection from impure thoughts, protection from moral degeneration and, crucially, protection from their own bodies, the very potential of their personal physicality. What this equally obsessive moral crusade represents is a politics of denial. It ensures that children, systematically and institutionally, are denied access to information and knowledge concerning their physical and sexual development and its broader social and cultural context.

While politicians and media commentators appear to revel in the opportunity to pontificate over declining moral standards, regularly proclaiming what constitutes the 'best interests' of children and young people, there is a notable silence in the public domain concerning their education in sexuality. As the emotional complexity of developing physicality and sexual awareness impacts on the lives of young people, the deeply personal issues and the struggle for understanding are diverted to the private domain. The family becomes the primary site for moral guidance and sexual understanding. Apart from the mass of evidence which demonstrates the problems associated with so-called parental guidance, the belief that the family constitutes a safe haven for children within which they can build relationships with adults based on trust, understanding and integrity is a misplaced act of faith. For, it is within the family and its extended adult network that children are most at risk from physical abuse and sexual exploitation. The abuse of children, pre-eminently a dehumanizing extension of father-right, cuts across societal divisions of class, ethnicity, culture and religion. It is both endemic and destructive, yet regularly normalized.

While the media has remained in hot pursuit of ritual abuse it has all but ignored ritualized abuse. It is only when cases of extreme abuse come to the fore, such as the 1995 trial of Rosemary West, that the possibility is entertained that there are many secrets, maybe not so extreme, hidden behind the closed doors of apparently well-functioning families. These fleeting thoughts pass with relief as the exceptional cruelty at the heart of such cases is interpreted as a reliable indicator that the ritualizing of sexual abuse is, equally, an aberration. And so, politicians, feature writers and 'informed' commentators, displaying a remarkable misreading of history, hark back to a 'golden age' of the family untroubled by abusing relationships, by disharmony or separation. It is portrayed as a period free of the necessity for child welfare professionals and uncontaminated by the unsettling agenda of feminist critiques. The battle cries of Thatcherism (return to Victorian Values) and of post-Thatcherism (Back to Basics), form part of an offensive against the assumed excesses of sexual promiscuity, familial permissiveness and declining morality.

Central to this offensive are claims that the 1960s spawned a sexual revolution among young people which involved unprecedented moral irresponsibility masquerading as sexual liberation. Under-age sex, premarital sex, multiple sexual partners, open homosexuality, bisexuality and transvestism are given as examples of unacceptable, perverse relations which together contributed to the demise of marriage and the family. What is maintained is that the self-styled 'liberationists' have had an undue influence on successive generations through weak parenting, divorce, single parenting, popular culture, professional ideologies and so on. It is the ground that they are assumed to occupy which has to be reclaimed in the reaffirmation of *basics*. While the issue is conceived and addressed as one of high moral values, the political reality is moral fundamentalism, incorporating an ideological backlash against feminism, homosexuality and any individuals or groups whose lifestyles challenge, or present alternatives to, the heterosexual family unit. Focusing particularly on children and young people, the public and highly publicized debate has addressed sexuality almost exclusively in terms of moral degeneracy, social contagion and the need to win their hearts and minds. This is a remarkable irony given the media's collusion, if not open advocacy, of sexual representation dominated by fantasies of sex, violence and degradation.

'She Devils' and Morality Panics

Once the academic and political critiques central to the emergence and consolidation of contemporary feminism began to have an impact on state policy, a backlash was inevitable (Coppock, Haydon and Richter, 1995). This has been the case particularly with those policies relating to the socialization and schooling of children and young people. During the 1970s a series of influential critiques developed which examined all aspects of the school process, including the formal and hidden curriculum, demonstrating the gender divide and its attendant hierarchy dominant in British schooling, its policies and practices. The media, political commentators and politicians seized on any specific cases or instances which they considered indicated the 'threat' of feminism to established order politics. Such stories had added value if they could be associated, however indirectly, with the personal sexual politics or assumed self-interest of those involved. In 1978 a deputy headteacher of a Hertfordshire village school, not the most likely location for a national debate over gender and education, became the focus of the much broader controversy.

Spare Rib was due to publish a special edition on sexism in schools and the deputy headteacher, Sally Shave, contributed an article. Prior to publication, the *Daily Express* covered the story with a major feature headlined 'Boys will be Boys'. In its editorial it stated: 'If Sally Shave, who is responsible for little children, does not mind them growing up neither men nor women, the sooner she turns her talents to working a capstan lathe or a manicurist's scissors the better' (Hemmings, 1980:168). Sally Shave's sexual politics were on the line leading to further criticism from parents, governors and journalists, none of whom had read her article. It was pointed out by governors that she always wore jeans to work and actively encouraged girls to wear trousers. The headteacher told her that she was, 'unwise to go so openly to the local pub with her "friends" and that, although he wasn't prejudiced, the village was not ready for people of her sort' (1980:169). A woman journalist, writing in the *Evening News*, accused her of propagating 'pernicious rubbish', and asked 'why Hertfordshire's education authorities allow her to practise her half-baked theories' (Hemmings, 1980:169). This was a clear attempt to have her disciplined or even dismissed from her post.

Within a week the *Sunday Express* projected the attack onto a broader terrain:

> Those teachers who as reported last week are trying to blur the distinction between boys and girls have a lot to learn. The trouble with these fanatical reformers like these non-sexist nuts is that they throw the baby out with the bath water and in their fervour to sweep away everything that is bad about discrimination, they sweep away everything that is good too. Equal opportunity is one thing because it offers choice. Being bulldozed into total sameness is quite another. If the non-sexist lot had their way, girls would be made to feel inadequate if they follow their age-old instincts to attract a mate, set up home, have babies and devote their life to looking after all three. This is not imposed upon them. It is as natural in girls as in a plant or a robin (Hemmings, 1980:170).

The fragility of gender and sexual relations is transparent in this response. It indicates a paranoia within patriarchal relations, that in challenging sexism within schools, girls will lose their 'natural' sexuality, deny their 'age-old instincts' and the social and biological imperatives of reproduction will be destroyed. The message was clear: that feminist critiques ('fanatical'; 'non-sexist nuts') were intent on denying girls their natural instincts and, therefore, those who proclaimed anti-sexist policies and practices were themselves unnatural or abnormal. The underlying inference was that Sally Shave was a lesbian intent on corrupting sound heterosexual socialization processes.

Such aggressive press coverage of sexuality, particularly its supposed concern with the relationship between 'adequate' motherhood and 'questionable' sexuality, dominated the regular features written on the women's peace camp at Greenham Common. The twin themes were those of the 'irresponsible mother' and the 'corruptibility' of the children, the former placing protest before family. 'What sort of women', demanded the *Daily Express* (9 March 1983), 'expose themselves to conditions like they are living in, and subject their children to the same thing?' In profiling one leading campaigner, Helen John, the *Daily Express* already had delivered its answer, condemning her as 'a woman and mother who has repudiated womanhood and motherhood in the name of sterile and arid feminism which is an insult to her sex and to humanity' (*Daily Express*, 10 January 1983).

The implied threat of the all-women peace camp as a suitable place for children was made explicit with the disclosure that at least one woman was living at the camp with her child and her lesbian lover. The story was irresistible and a *Daily Express* reporter, Sara Bond, went 'undercover' to write it. Predictably she revealed 'exclusively' that lesbians dominated the camp:

... striding the camp with their butch haircuts, boots and boilersuits. They flaunt their sexuality, boast about it, joke about it ... I became annoyed at the way doting couples sat around the camp fire kissing and caressing. A lot of women 'go gay' after arriving at the camp. With no men around they have to turn to each other for comfort. Other lesbians masquerade as peace women and go to Greenham just for sex ... (*Daily Express*, 10 April 1984).

This report 'from the front-line' not only set the seal on the relationship between the denial of motherhood and lesbian sexuality as unnatural and abnormal but it also represented the camp as a predatory environment of social contagion, a place of physical and psychological risk for children. These powerful images have remained significant and dominant, mobilized at every opportunity to defend heterosexuality, marriage and the family against the perceived onslaught of alternative sexualities, sexual preference and orientation. Since Greenham this has included: the near-hysterical debate over Section 28 (discussed later); HIV/AIDS policies; sexuality and the Armed Forces/ Anglican Church; the age of consent debate; homosexual/lesbian rights to foster or adopt children. The issue of sexuality in the context of sex education has been one of the most volatile sites of the debate.

In 1994 a series of unrelated events illustrated this volatility, providing renewed opportunities for the messages of moral fundamentalism to dominate the media. A Hackney primary school headteacher, Jane Brown, refused the offer of subsidized seats for her pupils to see a Royal Opera House production of Shakespeare's *Romeo and Juliet*. Her decision involved a complex mix of economic, staffing and curriculum issues. But she also indicated her concern about the ballet's underage sex, violence and heterosexism. Further, she voiced her professional judgment that books, films and theatre should reflect diverse sexualities and not be restricted to heterosexual culture.

The media instantly focused on the issue of sexuality and heterosexism, condemning Jane Brown without reference to her other concerns. John Patten, then Secretary of State for Education, stated that the decision was 'crackpot' reflecting 'the damaging effects of creeping political correctness' (*The Times*, 20 January 1994). The Chair of the Local Education Authority described it as 'an act of ideological idiocy and cultural philistinism' (*The Times*, 20 January 1994) which denied equal opportunities to children. Within hours of the story breaking a headteacher with an exemplary track record was pressured into making a public apology, 'forced to say something she did not believe' (Campbell, 1995:18) and 'publicly humiliated for national TV' (Radford, 1995–96:5). Bea Campbell commented that one of Britain's more progressive education authorities, with a prominent black educationalist as its director, 'was prepared to sacrifice a successful school and deliver its lesbian head to its own mortal enemies' (1995–6:20).

Inevitably, Jane Brown's sexuality, her personal life and relationships, were elevated to a matter of national significance. The open agenda, as at

Greenham, was whether a lesbian was a fit and proper person to manage a primary school. How could she have been appointed in the first place? Within days the press delivered its answer. Her partner, forced into hiding by the intrusion of insistent journalists, was named (and photographed) as being the acting chair of the school governors at the time of Jane Brown's appointment. The allegations, later shown to be false, were that she was in a relationship with the acting chair at the time of the appointment and that she had been coached for the post. While a school governors' inquiry fully exonerated Jane Brown, and a subsequent OFSTED report on the school was highly complimentary of the standard of education provided, the damage had been done. Yet again, a highly skilled woman had been vilified not only for her anti-sexist principles but also for her lifestyle, relationships and sexuality.

Within weeks a public health nurse, Sue Brady, was also forced into hiding. During a sex education class at a Leeds primary school she had answered questions about oral sex. Within hours of the initial publicity the headteacher made a public apology for what amounted to an 'error of judgment' (*Guardian*, 24 March 1994). David Blunkett, Shadow Education Secretary, condemned Sue Brady for 'crass and inappropriate provision of sex education' (*Guardian*, 26 April 1994). Journalists descended on the school and on her home, widely reporting that classroom discussions had centred on 'Mars Bars parties'. John Patten was quoted as being 'incensed' by the incident: 'I hope that I am never again faced with the sort of reports that I have had over the past 24 hours' (*Guardian*, 26 April 1994). Sue Brady, however, put the issue into context:

> Sometimes you get one or two streetwise children who try to shock, who will try to test you out. My belief is, rather than having children going out into the playground and getting a perverted and wrong description about something, I would prefer to tell them, in a sensitive way, the true facts ... I've become a pawn in a political game (*Observer*, 27 March 1994).

Married with children, Sue Brady experienced none of the public scrutiny over her personal life or sexuality to which Jane Brown had been subjected. What was brought into question was her professional judgment. Giving sensitive and informed answers to questions asked by 11-year-olds was roundly condemned as inappropriate and irresponsible, potentially perverting or contaminating their sexual innocence. Straight answers to straight questions was also the intention of the Health Education Authority's booklet, *Your Pocket Guide to Sex*, dismissed by then Health Minister, Brian Mawhinney, as 'smutty' and pulped before distribution (*Guardian*, 26 April 1994). This sequence of events resulted in a renewed reluctance within schools to become involved in projects relating to sex education. In April 1994, for example, an education theatre company had all its bookings cancelled because its production promoted safer sex. Ceri Hutton, of the National AIDS Trust, stated that teachers were frightened: 'They see the attacks ministers make on individual schools and they think "I don't want to let my school in for that sort of publicity"' (*Guardian*, 26 April 1994).

Constructing Childhood, Confining Sexuality

As established earlier, '*childhood*' and '*sexuality*' are contested terrains. Each has been the subject of intense academic, political and, particularly since 1945, professional debate. Taken together they share certain defining theoretical assumptions, specifically that they are linked to 'natural', developmental stages. Just as childhood is mapped according to physical growth and cognitive development, so sexuality is linked to physical and hormonal changes. Theoretical traditions within child development mirror popular assumptions, incorporating moral belief, that the successful journey through childhood is best guided by a nurturing motherhood and a disciplining fatherhood bound together within wholesome heterosexual family life. Similarly, while sexuality has been the site of theoretical, academic and political conflict, at the level of interpersonal relations and 'appropriate' knowledge it has been identified as a personal matter confined to the private domain of the family. In the broader debate, however, and reflective of the 'nature' versus 'nurture' dichotomy in child development, the key theoretical tensions have centred on the conflict between biological essentialists and social constructionists.

As Chapter 1 shows, the social and cultural construction of childhood, as it has developed to the present, was rooted in the political–economic conditions of mid-nineteenth century capitalism. It is important not to generalize a complex and volatile period, given the unpredictability of urban, industrial economic expansion and the emergent liberal state servicing the consolidating capitalist enterprise, but at the formal level protective legislation began to exclude children from productive work. Also significant was the fear, particularly among the ruling and mercantile classes, of the 'dangerous poor'. It was a dangerousness rooted not only in perceptions of revolutionary potential but also in associated social conditions particularly crime, public disorder, disease and moral degeneration (Stedman Jones, 1977). In this context medico-legal discourses underpinned public health interventions against 'dangerous sexualities' (Mort, 1987), with children and young people focal to such anxieties. Child protection, inevitably, was directed downwards from Victorian middle-class family values to the 'morally degenerate' and 'vice-ridden' poor. Church, the state and voluntary organizations combined to impose moral hygiene, using the language of physical disease, on the working classes. According to Weeks (1989:48) the 'conceptualisation of the separateness of children went hand in hand with the socially felt need to protect their purity and innocence.' What this incorporated was a process of regulation and control in which sexual relations were established as the preserve solely of adults. Childhood, as well as being a period of physical development, became socially constructed around dependency. As Jackson (1982:27) states, 'The anxiety and controversy surrounding the issue of children and sex must be seen in the context of this prolongation of childhood and the special status it is given.'

Part of that special status turned on the presumption of innocence and assumptions relating to protection. Foucault (1980:42) argues that children were both 'deemed incapable of self-expression' and 'immune to sexuality'. The threat of sexual corruption was the basis of institutional surveillance, regulation and control of the child. An example of this was the preoccupation with infantile masturbation which, by the mid-nineteenth century, had become 'a subject of obsessive concern', with the masturbator redefined as a perpetrator, 'the archetypal image of the sex deviant' (Weeks, 1989:49). Not only were children assumed to be in need of protection from the external forces of corruption but also from their own potentially 'wayward' desires. Young women's maturity was further regulated through clitoridectomy. While there is considerable debate over the extent to which children in pre-capitalist society were fully integrated into adult life, 'What cannot be disputed . . . is that within the capitalist epoch, concern over and surveillance of the sexual, emotional, social and physiological immaturity and lack of autonomy of those defined as within childhood has been progressive' (Evans, 1994:3).

Adolescence, closely associated with the biological/physiological developments around puberty, was eventually established as the intermediate stage between childhood and adulthood. Puberty's physical changes have constituted the key indicators of capability in terms of sexual relationships; the stage of puberty being a signifier of young people's potential awareness. Yet, as Jackson notes:

> individual sexual development does not seem to be affected by the rate of physical development as much as by social experience. There are many pre-pubescent thirteen year olds with well developed sexual interests and many sixteen year olds, well past puberty, who are far less mature in this respect (1982:105).

Goldman and Goldman (1982) reflect a range of research establishing that children are well aware of sex and sexuality prior to puberty, with adults, particularly parents, consistently underestimating children's capacity to understand and express sexual feelings and emotions. This is hardly surprising given the strength of the images and messages which contextualize their lives.

The central assumption governing adults' perceptions of children's capacity to understand sex, sexuality and sexual desire is that feelings and knowledge develop similarly to physicality. This biological essentialism, depicting adolescence as a natural period of progression, represents sexual awareness solely as heterosexual awareness. Consequently, 'naturalism' is not open to question but presented as a scientific discourse based on laws of nature. Within this discourse, male sexuality is naturally aggressive, predatory, powerful and unstable. Female sexuality, contrasting but complementary, is passive, submissive, servicing and pacifying. Whereas male sexuality has an instinctive capacity to be vagrant, women's sexuality is rooted in the instinct of motherhood and the biological imperative of reproduction. Left unchecked, male sexuality is both dangerous and volatile threatening the necessary morality and stability of social relations. Women's role, then, is to pacify and contain the powerful drives of men through heterosexual coupling and formalized marriage, regulated through legal discourse and the rule of law.

Griffin is emphatic in arguing that, 'Dominant discourses around sexuality still rely on the biological domain as a defining frame', with established mainstream analyses representing sexuality 'as a social institution in which heterosexuality was defined as normal, compulsory and a mark of maturity, resting on the representation of femininity and masculinity as complementary opposites' (1982:160). Jackson, while conceding that sexuality has a 'biological basis, in that nature has endowed us with a certain potential' argues that this 'does not make it biologically determined, or any more "natural" than other aspects of human behaviour' (1982:15). Her contention being that the endowment of potential 'does not dictate how we express (it) . . .' (1982:9). Clearly, sexuality is rooted in physicality manifested in the mechanics of arousal. But it is defined, contained, regulated and sanctioned within social, cultural and political contexts and their moral imperatives. Sexuality is neither monolithic nor universal but is socially constructed. As Weeks concludes:

> For, sex, despite its immediacy, is very much a cultural and a historic phenomenon. Whatever we like to think, we are not entirely free agents in this matter . . . Our choices are real and important . . . constrained by a very long and complex history and intricate power relations, which tell us, amongst other things, what is natural or unnatural, good or bad, permissible or impermissible (1993:2).

Jackson states, 'when we think we are simply "doing what comes naturally" our *sense of naturalness* derives not from biological facts but from socially constructed definitions of what is sexual' (1982:18). While these definitions are not totally determining they are significant in directing sexual behaviour and desire within set or established boundaries. They are, as Weeks states, 'constrained' by 'intricate power relations'. For Mort:

> power, or sets of power relations addressing sexuality, operate through a multiplicity of practices and apparatuses (. . . medicine, psychology, sociology, education) each of which is distinguished by its specific structures of regulation, which are non-reducible to a uniform or single strategy (1980:41).

Referring to Foucault's theorizing of discursive practices, Mort raises the significance of the specificity of 'institutional sites and social and cultural practices in the forms of knowledge–power relations which are integral to them, the types of subjects they construct and the strategies of resistance that are possible' (1980:42). The politics of reproduction and the institutionalization of the heterosexual family provide 'the particular "regime of truth" for the classification of other sexual practices' (1980:44) while the state 'is viewed as instrumental in the reproduction of dominant sexual ideologies' (1980:47). Sexualities other than heterosexuality, its only 'natural' objective being procreation, are rejected as deviant or perverse.

The centrality of reproduction in the delivery of 'appropriate' sexual knowledge or awareness to children and young people inevitably denies them their immediate feelings and emotions, their pleasure or desires. For young people experiencing such emotions or desires reproduction is a distant concept. They are expected to accept knowledge in a form restricted to one possible, and permissible, version of their future – marriage and parenthood. Their learning is predicated on abstinence and denial. As Segal (1990:160) argues, the 'continuing denial of childhood sexuality' coupled with the 'lack of adequate sex education' jeopardizes young people's potential in forming equal sexual relations with adults. For the categorization of childhood is 'over-rigid', restricting responsibility for caring, loving and physical relations until the magical, universal 'age-of-consent' is reached. Yet, 'Childhood sexuality . . . takes both active and passive forms, with multiple outlets and objects, most of them not congruent with the meanings attached to adult heterosexuality' (1990:211).

Measor (1989:42) interviewed girls in their first year at secondary school and found that 'their sexual world was covert, and mysterious; the way into it was not seen as open.' Lees (1993:116), from her interviews with young women, concludes that 'Active sexuality is only rendered safe when confined to marriage and wrapped in the aura of love', with marriage representing long-term 'economic and cultural security . . .'. She identifies the process of 'legitimacy of naturalness' (1993:132) through which 'girls reconcile the discrepancy between their knowledge of marriage and the universal expectation that that was their natural destiny' (1993:133). For girls, the endurance of menstruation, the clear indication and reminder that biology can feel like destiny with its direct link to reproduction, is sharpened by the subordinating attention from boys. As Lees shows, girls do not even have to be sexually active to be ascribed a negative reputation. 'The only security girls have against bad reputations is to confine themselves to the "protection" of one partner . . . [involving] dependency and loss of autonomy precisely because women's position in the family is subordinate and unequal' (1993:29).

The denial of young women's active sexuality is not just a personal issue, because structurally it 'reflects unfair power relations between the sexes' (1993:62). As femininity is subordinated to masculinity within patriarchies it is the agenda of 'becoming sexual' which girls and boys, young women and young men, have to negotiate. Connell, Radican and Martin reflect that masculinity, despite what male bravura represents, is not constituted in isolation but 'in relation to femininity, in the context of an over-arching structure of gender relations' (1987:6). In this context hegemonic masculinity labels and names the sexuality of girls but its expression, in public displays of misogyny and homophobia, can hide the private struggles which boys experience around sensitivity and personal vulnerability. As Mac an Ghaill's (1994) work with boys in a secondary school shows, while 'specific gender regimes' operate and are institutionalized, what prevails 'is a picture of complex inner-dramas of individual insecurity and low self-esteem' (1994:102). His in-depth analysis of the process of 'sexualization', as boys negotiate maleness/masculinity and experience the transition into 'manhood', challenges the false universalism of earlier work, revealing the complexities and contingencies of gender formation.

This process is mediated not only by the deeply personal world of self-identity and self-esteem but also by the structural and cultural imperatives of class and race. Mac an Ghaill concludes that 'misogyny, homophobia, heterosexism and racism are not passively inherited in a unitary or total way' (1994:179). Griffin makes a similar point in reflecting on her research with girls:

> All young women face pressures to move down the 'straight and narrow' path of heterosexuality, marriage and motherhood (in that order), but such pressures are experienced and negotiated in racialized and class-specific ways which also use notions of 'normality' and 'disability' to police the transition to adulthood. The voices of young women are seldom heard within the academic, clinical or judicio-legal literatures on 'premarital adolescent heterosexual intercourse', especially if they are working-class, Black and/or young women with disabilities (1993:241).

As the previous discussion indicates, childhood has been typified in popular, academic and professional discourses as 'incorrupt but corruptible, requiring family and educational institutions to preserve its innocence and purity en route to adulthood' (Evans, 1994:3). Given that the 'powerful definers' within these institutional discourses have trodden the route to adulthood it is difficult to accept the naïveté implicit in such assumptions. For they are aware that childhood experiences are informed and misinformed by sexual imagery, curiosity and half-truths. Both Wolpe (1988) and Mac an Ghaill (1994) demonstrate, through their closely-observed and collaborative research with young people, that parents provide minimal sex education. What little is discussed concentrates on biological reproduction solely in the context of heterosexist assumptions of male dominance and patriarchal power. Within schools, Wolpe (1988:100) notes that while 'sexual issues are ever present' they are 'not necessarily recognised as such by teachers'. As has been established, sexuality permeates the school environment but the ideology of 'childhood innocence' rejects schools as cultural sites where emergent sexual identities are formed, reproduced and lived. Also denied is the active engagement of children and young people in the formation of their sexual identities. Thus schools are desexualized (Epstein and Johnson, 1994). Mac an Ghaill notes:

Ironically, at a time of much pedagogical rhetoric about student-centred teaching approaches and cross-curricular initiatives, there appears to be little movement among policy makers or within schools to design whole-school programmes of effective sex education that starts with the students' experiences and needs (1994:156).

It is because such experiences and needs are denied legitimacy that appropriate programmes fail to emerge. What is taught reflects a narrow but purposeful commitment to the mechanics and functions of biological reproduction, 'often little more than teaching about biology, reproduction and virology' (Haffner, 1992:vii). As Griffin (1993:160) argues, 'Dominant discourses around sexuality still rely on the biological domain as the defining frame', and this domain provides a veneer of 'scientism'. Consequently the curriculum restricts consideration of sexuality to that of heterosexual relations as 'normal, compulsory and a mark of maturity' (1993:160), but contained within the social institutions of marriage and the family. Similarly, Sears (1992:7) maintains that 'sexuality education' in the USA is primarily 'an instrument of sexual and social control', its effectiveness judged on the successful regulation of sexual behaviour. As Thomson argues:

State schools not only provide an environment enabling universal access to the under-16 'population', but schools are also public arenas in which hegemonic or 'official' representations of personal and public morality are expressed. As such schools are key sites for both social engineering and control (1993:220).

It is within this regulatory context that children and young people learn to 'weigh the costs and benefits of particular sexual behaviour' with primary emphasis placed on 'the prevention of adolescent heterosexual coital activity' (Sears, 1992:13). Further, as Measor states, what is provided by teachers is 'derived from their own culture and from their adult status' (quoted in Mac an Ghaill, 1994:156).

According to Haffner, less than 10 per cent of children in the USA receive comprehensive sexuality education from nursery through to adulthood. She concludes:

the official curriculum teaches a reproductive heterosexuality, removed from discussions of gender politics, violence, economics and even pleasure. Programs are often based on a model that assumes all children live in two-parent family middle-class homes and will grow up to be monogamous, married for life, heterosexual adults (1992:vii).

Sears states that 'schools socialize boys and girls into their presumed hetero-sexual identity' (1992:146). Griffin, in her comparative analysis of youth sexu-ality in the USA and UK concludes that 'young people are presumed to be heterosexual until otherwise indicated, and the mark of "mature" sexuality is taken to be the first experience of heterosexual intercourse, specifically penetration' (1993:167). Inevitably, any expression of sexuality other than penetrative heterosexual sex is 'rendered invisible (lesbianism, celibacy) or criminal (gay male sexuality)...' (1993:168). On this basis, what Sears (1992:13) refers to as the 'language of sexual intimacy, the fluidity of sexuality, and the creativity of human sexual responses' are rendered unnatural, abnor-mal and immoral by the sex/sexuality education curriculum. And, as Mac an Ghaill has found, school students have views on this systematic denial:

> In criticizing conventional programmes of sex education, the stu-dents are challenging the structures and practices involved in the desexualization of school life, in which not only is homosexuality excluded but by sleight of hand all aspects of sexuality other than the institutional form of the monogamous family structure is written out of the curriculum (1994:158).

The process of 'desexualization' is not only passive and Whatley argues persuasively that teachers 'self censor' as a direct result of the 'conservative shift in the debates around sexuality education due to the constant attacks from the New Right' (1992:79). As discussed earlier, teachers do not want to draw attention to their schools even though, as Lees found, 'some teachers quietly broadened sex education to include real issues facing young people, including questions of sexual orientation' (1993:221). The impact of the New Right, the self-proclaimed 'moral majority' and the religious fundamentalists cannot be over-stated.

Feeding the Myths, Forging the Policies

In the UK public anxiety over moral degeneracy was fuelled by the Thatcherite project within the New Right during the late 1970s and early 1980s. It was an appeal to public indignation founded on three assumptions, paraded as facts. These were: the demise of the traditional family unit (through divorce/lone mothers/cohabitation); the legacy of the permissiveness of the late 1960s/early 1970s; the threat of sexual diversity posed by the lesbian and gay movement. The growth of feminism was targeted specifically as re-sponsible for giving academic and political credibility to these trends through its challenge to gender demarcation and compulsory heterosexuality. Also targeted were those local authorities and public institutions which had adopted equal opportunities policies and programmes, and had founded specialist research, information and campaign units. As the first Thatcher

Government came to power in 1979, partly on a platform of affirming a renewed morality, many local authorities, most ostensibly the Greater London Council, were initiating provision which reflected sexually diverse constituencies. It was a collision course which became immediately apparent in highly publicized disputes over sex education in London schools. Simply by advocating more open discussion in schools over homosexuality and lesbianism, the charge of 'gay lessons' was laid at the door of the Inner London Education Authority (Holly, 1989).

The political tensions which followed the initial attacks on local authorities and schools, and the aim of the traditionalists to '(establish) . . . the agenda of sexuality teaching inside the boundaries set by heterosexual familialism' (Redman, 1994:132), were derived in several distinct, but related, issues. These were: the onset of HIV/AIDS and the media-hyped panic over health education; children's rights of access to information (the Gillick Case); new restraints on teaching and information concerning sexuality (Section 28); the transfer of responsibility for sex education to school governing bodies (1986 Education (No 2) Act). For, as Haffner reflects, 'Recognising that they have lost the battle to prevent sexuality education, opposition groups now focus upon promoting their own brand of sexuality education, based on teaching moral absolutes and withholding information from children' (1992:viii). The issue of access to appropriate information is well-illustrated by the Gillick Case.

Gillick

In 1981 Victoria Gillick, a mother who publicly proclaimed her religious/moral conviction, demanded guarantees from her local authority that girls under 16 would be refused contraception or abortion without parental knowledge or consent. The local authority refused and this led to a protracted legal battle ending in 1986 with a House of Lords judgment. Gillick's position was that by prescribing contraceptives a doctor would increase the likelihood of under-age sexual intercourse. She maintained that this amounted to 'promoting, encouraging and facilitating' unlawful sexual intercourse in contravention of the 1956 Sexual Offences Act, S 28(1). Eight of the nine judges rejected the argument, finding that a doctor's intention would be to protect from pregnancy rather than to promote or encourage sexual intercourse. They ruled that, 'while it should be most unusual for a doctor to provide such a service to a child under 16 without parental knowledge or consent, there were circumstances . . . where he or she would be justified in doing so' (Department of Education and Science, 1987:5). The judgment, however, led to confusion:

> a doctor may treat a girl under 16 regarding birth control without her parents' knowledge or consent provided that i) it is in her best interests; ii) she will understand the advice; iii) she cannot be persuaded to tell her parents; iv) without advice or treatment her health

would suffer; v) she would begin or continue her sexual activity any way. This compromise is confusing for many: medical practitioners must proceed with caution, adolescents are unclear and parents are unsure (Hudson and Ineichen, 1991:34).

The 1987 Department of Education and Science (DES) Circular, *Sex Education at School*, stated that the ruling was limited to the 'nature and context of medical advice and treatment in connection with the supply and use of contraceptive devices', but that there was 'no parallel in school education' (DES, 1987:5). Teachers approached about such matters were advised to refer the child to his or her parents and to warn the child of risks if it was considered that he or she was in moral or physical danger, or in breach of the law. The Circular, however, left teachers with a serious dilemma:

> Whether the teacher should take the matter further, by informing the head teacher, and whether the head teacher should consider involv-ing the pupil's parents, the specialist support services, or the local education authority, will depend on the particular circumstances in-volved and the professional judgment of the staff (DES, 1987:5).

Yet, in a previous paragraph, the Circular warned that giving advice without parental knowledge and consent could, 'depending on the circum-stances, amount to a criminal offence' (DES, 1987:5). In contrast to the ambi-guity of the Circular, Bainham (1989:186) argues that the Gillick judgment 'supports rather than detracts from the legal entitlement of mature adoles-cents to approach professionals for advice' including a 'strong case for compul-sory sex education embracing reproductive biology, advice on contraception and discussion of the role of sexual activity within the context of caring relationships and family life.' Bainham argues that compulsion is the only means through which the rights of school children to accurate knowledge concerning sexual relationships can be achieved.

While Bainham's position has been endorsed by others (see NAPCE, 1993), the confusion within the 1987 Circular was extended by subsequent legislation and directives, promoting a climate of fear within schools. The 1994 DFE Circular, *Sex Education in Schools* states:

> The general rule must be that giving an individual pupil advice on such matters without parental knowledge or consent would be an inappropriate exercise of a teacher's professional responsibilities. Teachers are not health professionals, and the legal position of a teacher giving advice in such circumstances has never been tested in the courts (DFE, 1994:14).

Again, the route from teacher to headteacher to parents, thus breaching confidentiality, is prescribed but there is no indication of the legal boundaries within which teachers should give advice or support. The National Children's Bureau (NCB) advises that it is 'a matter of professional judgment for a teacher whether he or she should indicate to a child that information could be offered confidentially and whether such confidence could be maintained having heard the information' (NCB, 1994). The NCB is also confident that teachers giving contraceptive advice to under 16s, acting in the best interests of the child, probably would not be criminally prosecuted. Stevenson argues that the DFE directive denying teachers the potential to give contraceptive advice to under 16s without parental knowledge or consent, on the basis that it constitutes an 'inappropriate exercise of a teacher's professional responsibilities', contradicts the Government White Paper, *The Health of the Nation*, which prioritizes a reduction in 'under-age conceptions' through health and sex education programmes (1994:12).

The House of Lords' ruling, followed by circulars and legislation, together reflect a political compromise which has resulted in ambiguity for those delivering sex education. While it is unlikely that prosecutions would follow 'inappropriate advice', unless children had been formally withdrawn from sex education classes, there are no guarantees. Inevitably, as discussed earlier, this has led to self-censorship with teachers reluctant to overstep a mark which is yet to be drawn. The climate of fear governing sex education in schools, both formal and informal, has not been restricted to the debate over Gillick. Alongside this debate has been the contested area of sexuality and diversity. As Watney (1991:390) states, 'no area of social life has been subjected to a more violent ideological contestation in the modern period than sex education and the whole vexed question of homosexuality in schools' (1991:390).

HIV/AIDS

The climate in which sexuality education came to be debated during the 1980s grew increasingly hostile as a buoyant and bullish Thatcherism occupied, virtually unopposed, the moral high ground. Its political consolidation owed much to ideological successes, particularly convincing the electorate that by undermining local government, and in the case of the GLC its abolition, people would be freed from the vagaries and interventions of local politics. Targeted were those councils which had pioneered and developed provision for oppressed, identifiable groups. With the Tory press unrelenting in its search for 'loony left' stories from within local authorities, fabricating what it could not find (Hollingsworth, 1986; Taylor, 1992), sexuality became a key focus. Local government support for gay and lesbian initiatives was used as a metaphor for a sick society in moral decline. This vitriolic and deeply hypocritical attack from the New Right, whose spin-doctors had hijacked the twin concepts of freedom and liberty, coincided with the moral panic over HIV/AIDS.

HIV/AIDS, and the medico-legal discourses which dominated public debate, was promoted as the 'gay plague'. The denigration of the physical body, relentlessly manifested in AIDS, was cruelly mobilized as testimony to the degeneration of the social body. Biological contagion was promoted as synonymous with social contagion and the guilty parties were those who defended and promoted 'dangerous sexualities'. So powerful was the backlash against homosexuality that Patricia Hewitt, formerly General Secretary of the National Council for Civil Liberties and at the time the Labour Party leader's press secretary, wrote in a private letter that the 'lesbian and gay rights issue is costing us dear amongst pensioners' (*Capital Gay*, 13 March 1987; *The Guardian*, 7 March 1987). In the same month Geoffrey Dickens, a vocal Conservative backbencher, was unequivocal in his position:

> What we should be saying is: 'Look, I'm afraid this sort of behaviour is totally unacceptable. You're putting *your nation at risk* by your behaviour. We're not going to have this in the future. And that's why we're legislating to make this a crime once again (in Jeffery-Poulter, 1991:213).

As Griffin concludes:

> The panic over HIV and AIDS crystallised these various elements, concentrating on gay male sexuality, injecting drug users, and young people's supposedly promiscuous sexual practices (both heterosexual and homosexual), all of which were presumed to pose serious threats to the heterosexual family norm (1993:160).

In this context the Conservative Government proposed to amend local government legislation, ostensibly to protect children and young people against homosexuality but in reality to attack and regulate diversity and preference. As Smith argues, it was the central conviction of the moral traditionalists that 'homosexuality must be displaced from the childhood space in which "true" sexuality is carefully nurtured: if homosexuality is to emerge it must do so later' (1995:309). In May 1986 the tabloid press picked up a story from Islington concerning a book, *Jenny Lives with Eric and Martin*, held at a teachers' resource centre. Within days, ill-informed coverage reflected sensationalist headlines: homosexuals were accused of 'propagating' their 'peculiar practices at the public expense' (*Sunday Mirror*, 3 May 1986); 'VILE BOOK IN SCHOOL' (*Sun*, 6 May 1986); 'SCANDAL OF GAY PORN BOOKS READ IN SCHOOLS' (*Today*, 7 May 1986). The die was cast as the book became a vehicle for the moralists who sought to use the proposed Education Bill to regulate sex education. Baroness Cox pronounced, without any evidence, that 'in this age of AIDS' it was beyond belief that local authorities and their teachers were 'promoting gay issues in the curriculum' (quoted in Jeffery-Poulter, 1991:208). On 8 December 1987, at the Committee stage of the proposed Local Government Bill, an amendment was introduced forbidding local authorities to promote homosexuality or publish material for the promotion of homosexuality or to promote the teaching in any maintained school of the acceptability of homosexuality as a *pretended family relationship*. Eventually to become Section 28, initially Clause 28, this amendment became the focus of one of the most orchestrated and fierce examples of the backlash against sexual diversity.

Section 28

The 1988 Local Government Act introduced three key statutory limitations on local authorities: no intentional promotion of homosexuality; no publication of material intended to promote homosexuality; no teaching in maintained schools of the acceptability of homosexuality as a pretended family relationship. Undoubtedly children and young people were the focus of attention. Margaret Thatcher stated that 'children who need to be taught to respect traditional moral values are being taught that they have an inalienable right to be gay' (in Evans, 1989:74). Michael Howard, later to become Home Secretary, argued that parents 'have become increasingly concerned about public money being used in that way to influence the attitudes and behaviour of impressionable young people' (in Thomas and Costigan, 1990:9). Terry Dicks MP spoke for many on the Conservative right when he ranted, 'These homosexuals should take their handbags and lipsticks elsewhere . . . God help any of them who taught such filth to my grandchild in school' (quoted in *Sun*, 17 December 1987). Another vocal Conservative MP, Jill Knight, on hearing that Section 28 did not extend to school governors or teachers, stated that there was some mistake for, 'The major point of it was to protect children in schools from having homosexuality thrust upon them' (in Durham, 1991:118).

The portrayal of heterosexuality as 'vulnerable' and homosexuality as a powerful, destructive force demonstrated the assumed fragility of established order sexuality. Watney (1991) argues that, in the process of protecting young people from the 'promotion' of sexuality, there was no consideration of the position of gay teachers or students. Neither was there any consideration of children and young people with same sex parents, or with gay relatives or friends. Publicly, and without qualification, such families were condemned and dismissed as 'pretended'. This was 'Parliament's disapprobation of families in which adults are gay' (Thomas and Costigan, 1990:14). Wilton (1995) argues that Section 28 represented the overt heterosexualization of the family and Evans (1995) identifies its impact as both symbolic and ideological, bringing stringent self-regulation and censorship in institutional practices. While the statutory requirements concerning promotion, according to Lord Gifford (Colvin, 1989), remain legally unworkable, they had 'the insidious effect of constructing teachers as the potential corrupters of young people . . . frightening teachers from saying what they thought was sensible and right out of fear of losing their jobs' (Thomson, 1993:225).

The legacy of Section 28 became evident in the subsequent sex education legislation. Homosexuality, together with contraception, abortion, child abuse and pornography were deemed 'sensitive issues'. This emphasizes the negative construction of homosexuality, a far cry from 'an approach that would genuinely seek to integrate the reality of gay and lesbian sexuality into the taken-for-granted life of the school as just one more aspect of school diversity' (Redman, 1994:133). The DFE Circular on Sex Education (DFE, 1994:19) affirms Section 28 but maintains the climate of confusion and fear. While noting that the prohibitive intent of Section 28 is directed towards 'activities of local authorities themselves' and is 'distinct from the activities of the governing bodies and staff of schools' (DFE, 1994:14), its presence in the circular acts as a warning, inevitably encouraging the mistaken assumption that it could apply to governors' policies and teachers' practices. Inevitably, it 'feeds the myth that educating the young and homosexuality are incompatible' (Epstein and Johnson, 1994:224).

The 1994 DFE Circular also confirmed Section 46 of the 1986 Education Act, that all parties should ensure that sex education in schools 'is given in such a manner as to encourage those pupils to have due regard to moral considerations and the value of family life' (DFE, 1994:18). It continues:

> Pupils should accordingly be encouraged to appreciate the value of stable family life, marriage and the responsibilities of parenthood. They should be helped to consider the importance of self-restraint, dignity, respect for themselves and others, acceptance of responsibility, sensitivity towards the needs of others, loyalty and fidelity (1994:6).

If the term *promotion* is at all appropriate it relates to the boundaries drawn around heterosexuality within the context of biological reproduction and the nuclear family. As Stevenson argues, limitations are placed on 'young people's access to a range of diverse information', the assumption being that they are 'incapable of making their own decisions about the sexual practices and lifestyles most appropriate to their lives' (1994:11). This institutional denial of access has been achieved through guidelines and directives which have no statutory status yet which have been interpreted as regulatory and defining by many governors and teachers. What this process has resulted in is a 'climate in which schools tread with extreme caution', with 'heterosexual familialism ... actively and passively presented by schools as an unproblematic social and moral norm' (Redman, 1994:133) extending beyond the formal sex education curriculum to the hidden curriculum.

While school governors and teachers are afforded some discretion in developing sex education policy and content, the 1993 Education Act enables parents to withdraw children from classes other than those within the National Curriculum. The latter is restricted entirely to biological reproduction within the science curriculum. Once again, the rights of the child or young person are determined by the rights of the parent or adult. There was no consultation with children and young people concerning the DFE guidelines and, in terms of legislation, the 1993 Education Act reflects a 'sorry tradition of muddled official thinking and proscriptive policy-making when what is needed is clear sighted innovation and a willingness to address real needs' (Redman, 1994:148).

Age of Consent

In 1994 the debate over sexuality and young people's rights was renewed. Reforms of the age of consent for homosexual acts between consenting males were proposed and debated within the context of the Criminal Justice and Public Order Bill. The 1967 Sexual Offences Act set the age of consent for homosexuals at 21, whereas for heterosexuals it was set at 16. A common age of consent had been a key campaigning objective of gay groups throughout the 1970s and 1980s (see Smith, 1995). Eventually, Parliament decided on a compromise, to reduce the age of consent for homosexual relations in private to 18, thereby legislating to retain discrimination. Again, the debate was dominated by the issue of 'protection', presented as necessary not only for 'vulnerable' young boys who lacked maturity and had no fixed sexuality, but also for those whose sexuality was thought to be affirmed. Further, the reformists were committed to establishing and winning on the principle of equality rather than legitimizing homosexuality as equivalent to heterosexuality.

Edwina Currie, a Conservative MP and former minister, argued the case on the basis of human rights, equality before the law and the potential embarrassment of a defeat on the issue in the European Court. She used the concept of protection, but from a different perspective, arguing that the intimidatory and deterrent nature of the law was 'extremely damaging', inhibiting 'young men from seeking help, whether through counselling, health advice or sex education' (*Hansard*, 21 February 1994:75). Using a range of medical sources and evidence to support her contention that the criminalization of gay sex inhibited effective health education and appropriate healthcare, she asked, 'How can we advise young gay men about the dangers of AIDS, how can we talk to them straight about safer sex, when what they are doing is supposed to be strictly against the law?' (*Hansard*, 1994:78). Clearly the apparent progressive move towards reform was limited, being based primarily on the protection of young people's sexual, emotional and psychological health. Medical discourses still prevailed, even among the reformists, over alternative discourses which would guarantee and safeguard the rights of children to explore and express their sexuality openly, without fear of legal or institutional sanction. Even this was too much for the moralists, with Harry Greenway asking that the House of Commons 'protect the young men of the nation (*Hansard*, 1994:75) and Tony Marlow maintaining that what was being sought was the legalization of 'buggery of adolescent males' (*Hansard*, 1994:78).

The compromise was struck on the basis of two arguments. The first, put by Sir Anthony Durant and supported by the Archbishop of York, was that young men reach maturity at 18 and that they should be given a longer opportunity to assess the social consequences of a decision concerning homosexuality (*Hansard*, 1994:87–8). The second, put by Michael Howard, was that 'most parents hope and expect their sons to follow a heterosexual lifestyle and hope that in due course they will build a family of their own' (*Hansard*, 1994:95) and to lower the age of consent to 16 would put this process at risk given the 'consequences' of homosexual activities. He concluded:

> it would be wrong to ignore the instinctive and deeply held concern of many people that a decision to have homosexual sex is different from a decision to have heterosexual sex . . . we shall not offend against any fundamental or civil right if we continue to reflect in the criminal law a public understanding of the difference between homosexual activity and heterosexual activity (1994:96).

It is not surprising that such 'deeply held concern' exists within a society steeped in ignorance and homophobia. That it is 'instinctive', as opposed to socially and politically constructed, is unsustainable. Homosexual experiences prior to establishing the 'settled' relationships offered by heterosexuality are presented as the consequences of pressure and/or corruption from older, homosexual predators. This was a line adopted by Lady Olga Maitland in proposing that a 16-year-old boy 'troubled by his growing sexuality', 'unsettled and frightened of girls', could be 'strongly pressured by the gay lobby' and was in need of legal protection (*Hansard*, 1994:80). Michael Alison, MP, similarly argued that such young men could find their sexuality 'altered' and 'redirected' by a 'highly organised, self-conscious community' (*Hansard*, 1994:104). Consequently they would 'lose . . . the option of family life and *normal* parenthood' (*Hansard*, 1994:104, emphasis added).

Again the debate focused on the aberrant, as well as abhorrent, construction of homosexuality. Bill Walker demanded protection because homosexuality was 'neither normal or natural' (*Hansard*, 1994:78). Predictably, the Rev. Ian Paisley was uncompromising:

> As goes the family, so will go the nation . . . The *normal* sex act, within the marriage vow, bringing together male and female and producing offspring, is the *happy* way; it is the *divine* way; it is the *creative* way; and it is the *best* way . . . We should be trying to *save* young men and boys from going down the homosexual road. We should be bringing them to the joys of true marriage and raising a family. We should dedicate ourselves not to the destruction of young boys but to their deliverance. They need to be delivered (1994:14, emphasis added).

To that contribution, which also drew the distinction between 'living in normality' and 'in abnormality,' Sir Nicholas Fairbairn added 'heterosexual activity is normal and homosexual activity, putting your penis into another man's arsehole, is a perverse – . . .' (1994:98. He was interrupted).

Despite the level of hostility towards reform, it was agreed to lower the age of consent to 18. In reviewing this 'compromise', Smith (1995:31) considers that while the vote to lower the age to 16 was lost 'the argument appeared to have been won'. Yet much of the 1967 Sexual Offences Act, relating to 'gross indecency', the concept of 'private place' and the legacy of discrimination against homosexuality, remains untouched. Retaining a distinction between homosexual and heterosexual relations, and ensuring that distinction through differential legal ages of consent, was a reaffirmation of heterosexuality as *the* sexuality. While the protection of 'vulnerable' young men from their own developing sexuality, its identity and its relations, was the paramount objective to be achieved, the reduction in the age of consent by 3 years was a hollow victory.

In Whose Best Interest?

Each of the debates covered here, from Gillick through Section 28 to the age of consent, exemplifies the profound problems associated with establishing an alternative and relevant agenda for the rights of children and young people regarding knowledge of sex and sexuality. Access to appropriate and reliable information in the public, institutional sphere (schools, youth work, healthcare agencies) has been replaced by an act of faith in the effectiveness of the private domain of the family. Despite deepening concern over health-related issues, the continuing rise in teenage pregnancies and the paucity of sound and effective advice and counselling, a climate of fear pervades throughout those agencies with responsibilities for children and young people. For example, when Mac an Ghaill asked sixth-form and further education tutors if he could discuss 'masculinity' with their students he was told that homosexuality was an inappropriate topic, given the implications of Section 28. He concludes:

> Such self-surveillance has been the specific and frequently misunderstood hidden state agenda developed . . . with the emergence of the New Right and the New Right moralism . . . Implicit in the teachers' responses was the assumption that dominant forms of heterosexual masculinity are unproblematic (1994:155).

Mac an Ghaill's experiences identify a serious deficiency, not limited to schools and colleges, derived in a combination of ambivalence, misunderstanding and fear. What is available as information, advice or treatment services for children and young people falls far short of the provision necessary, let alone ideal. For Haffner adequate provision:

encompasses sexual knowledge, beliefs, attitudes, values, and behaviours . . . At its best, sexuality education is about social change – about helping to create a world where all people have the information and the rights to make responsible sexual choices – without regard to age, gender, socio-economic status, or sexual orientation (1992:vii).

The pockets of progress towards these ends, even the renaming of *sex* education as *sexuality* education, have been inhibited, if not curtailed, within the prevailing moral and political backlash. Social and cultural experiences and expressions of sexuality have been denied by the reaffirmation of biological determinism and medicalization. The recent evolution in sex education, strongly evident in successive DFE circulars, has been 'determined more by the consequences of moral panics than rationalisation' (Meredith in Thomson, 1993:231–2).

The denial of childhood sexuality is an essential component of the broader negation of children and young people as active citizens. The contradictions concerning their rights to consultation and expression are sharply evident in the interpretation of domestic legislation and international conventions. For example, the principle underpinning the 1989 Children Act, that the 'wishes and feelings of the child' (considered in terms of 'age' and 'understanding') should be sought, is not realized in sex/sexuality education policy or practice. The intention of the Act, to strike 'a new balance between family autonomy and the protection of children' actually limits the right to participation and consultation because adults, in both public and private spheres, are the sole definers of the criteria which establish 'appropriate age and understanding'. This is one of a range of examples which empowers adults (be they agency managers, school governors, teachers, youth workers, health workers) and gives them broad discretion to construct policy, establish need and give information/treatment.

The diminution of the rights of children and young people to receive appropriate sexuality education, conflicts with the UN Convention on the Rights of the Child, specifically 'Article 24.2(f)'s particular emphasis on developing preventive healthcare and family planning education' (CRDU, 1994:106). Article 13 states, 'the child shall have the right to freedom of expression; this right shall include freedom to seek, receive and impart information and ideas of all kinds . . .' To establish and protect this right children should be active participants in discussions and decisions which contextualize sexualities, including their own, within policy, curriculum and information provision. Further, Article 3 establishes the concept of the 'best interests of the child', declaring a duty of care and protection for children's 'well-being' and a duty of quality provision of appropriate services and facilities. Article 24 provides for the right to the 'highest level of healthcare possible and access to healthcare services', particularly preventive healthcare including family planning education and services. Taken together these provisions, defined and endorsed internationally, are systematically neglected within the UK, despite its ratification of the UN Convention in December 1991.

In January 1995 the UN Committee on the Rights of the Child directed 'several subjects of concern' towards the UK. One of the most serious was that the 'principle of best interests of the child appears not to be reflected in legislation such as health, education and social security' (para. 213). Unsurprisingly, the Committee was concerned that 'insufficient attention has been given to the right of the child to express his/her opinion', specifying the parental right to withdraw children from sex education classes. The Committee's concerns reflect many of the issues raised in this chapter. The infantilizing of children, sustaining childhood as a prolonged denial of personhood or citizenship, is particularly marked with regard to their developing sexualities. As the Children's Rights Office states, children's capacities are seriously underestimated and this 'sets up a self-conforming cycle' (CRO, 1995b:23). In protecting their innocence, children's experiences and competencies are neglected – with adults directing and determining their behaviour, choices, opportunities and potential. Denied independence, or the information and experiences necessary to develop their emerging sexualities, children and young people are made vulnerable.

The message from children and young people is clear. A 1994 Mori poll found that 82 per cent of 16–19 year olds interviewed considered the state had a role to play in providing full and appropriate information to young people, and 37 per cent considered that sex education in schools started too late (*Guardian*, 9 January 1994). A Health Education Authority survey in March 1994 found that 84 per cent of children polled considered it helpful to consult a teacher about contraception or related issues. But 64 per cent would not consult if they thought that parents would be informed. Two-thirds of the 87 local authorities surveyed by the Sex Education Forum (1992), however, indicated confusion and uncertainty over the function and content of sex education in their schools. A quarter of schools had no sex education policy, a problem highlighted by Haydon and Corteen (1996) in their research into primary school provision. Forty-six per cent of local authorities could not identify how many of their schools had policies. CRDU (1994) notes that only 56 per cent of health authorities are resourced to provide a Youth Advisory Service. There is clear evidence from this range of research that parental pressure, governors' disapproval, public disquiet and political controversy has undermined effective provision. Yet young people remain concerned about the lack of information and counselling provided around contraception, abortion, HIV/AIDS and sexualities.

Reflecting the concern of the UN Committee, the Children's Rights Development Unit (CRDU, 1994:105) concludes that 'appropriate, effective contraceptive and planning information and sex education is vital to the health of children and young people'. The UN Committee (CRO, 1995a, para 27:23–24) recommends that the provisions concerning best interests and consultation should be incorporated into UK administrative and legislative measures and policies. It requested 'further mechanisms' for the participation of children and young people in decisions, 'including within the family and the community'. The rights to consultation and to expression must move beyond health-related issues, however important they are, to enable children and young people to access information, advice, counselling and services with full confidentiality guaranteed. Sex education should be extended to sexuality education. It is only when children and young people can discuss, explore and understand the diversity of sexualities that homophobia, bigotry, exclusion and violence will be challenged. As Sanders and Spraggs (1989:17–18) conclude, the objectives should be to remove the 'isolation, fear and confusion' of young people, 'victimised and vulnerable' because of their perceived sexuality, and to enable them to 'think about their own and other people's sexual feelings' through discussing 'the diverse forms of sexuality and love within an honest and tolerant framework'.

Chapter 5

'Crisis' in the Classroom?

Deena Haydon

As the assumed 'crisis' in childhood is perceived and portrayed as deepening, so the two institutions most closely associated with children's lives – the family and the school – have become the primary targets for politicians, policy commentators and media editorial writers. Within popular discourse the images of children as unacceptably disruptive and disrespectful are matched by portrayals of schools infected by 'progressive' teaching methods and declining academic standards. Alleged 'scandals' such as that at William Tyndale Junior School during the mid-1970s, where staff were said to be in rebellion against governors, parents, the Local Education Authority (LEA) and politicians over curriculum content and classroom practice, are used to demonstrate chaos in classrooms and the education profession. As Chapter 2 shows, the much-hyped, mostly inaccurate, but highly publicized accounts of organized and collective violence by children at a Liverpool primary school were also immediately amplified as indicative of a 'crisis in our schools'. This was reminiscent of headlines such as 'Spare the Rod, Spoil the Child' which dominated coverage of the 1980–81 inner city disturbances. Throughout the 1980s and 1990s successive prime ministers and their education ministers have railed against 'leftie' teachers and their 'trendy' methods. The inevitable assumption, particularly evident in the political outbursts which followed the killing of James Bulger, has been that schools fail to provide children with appropriate knowledge, necessary skills, behavioural markers or moral standards. If there is something rotten in society, its roots have been traced to the modern classroom.

All positive indicators of developing, expanding and diversified educational opportunities have been brushed aside by ideological and political dogma, much of it originating with the emergence of the New Right in the late 1970s, whose rhetoric has been successfully mobilized as 'fact' based on analysis. The claims are that the achieved high standards of some postwar 'golden era' are in decline, particularly in literacy and numeracy. Young people are inadequately prepared for the world of work. Discipline, in many schools, has broken down with virtually no effective control or management of pupils. This has resulted in escalating truancy rates, school exclusions and outbreaks of serious violence in and around schools. Progressive teaching methods have given children free rein to question, doubt and challenge authority and, through mixed ability teaching, have reduced classes to the lowest common denominator. Comprehensivization has hindered the academic advancement of more able pupils while failing to provide vocational training for the less able.

More broadly, the claims extend to include academics, educational theorists and teacher trainers who are assumed to have undermined educational theory and practice through the active promotion of 'left-wing', 'child-centred' perspectives. This drive to revolutionize the classroom has been portrayed as having the active support of such contrasting bodies as trade unions, the inspectorate service and Department for Education (DFE) civil servants. Local authorities, particularly the former Inner London Education Authority (ILEA), have been identified as complicit in this challenge to the established order within British education. Outside schools, but evident in the communities they serve, has been the systematic 'breakdown of the family'. As Chapter 3 argues, this image has been all-pervasive and with regard to schools the portrayal has been that of declining parental support for education, ill-disciplined children and the absence of appropriate role models on whom to rely for the development of 'appropriate' moral values and behaviour. Finally, schools have been implicated in the rejection of Christian religion and an emphasis on secularism or pluralism. This, it is assumed, has undermined Christian values and their connection to 'British' culture and heritage.

The ideology of the New Right, beginning with the publication of the Black Papers on Education (Cox and Dyson, 1969a, 1969b, 1971) and the Gould Report's (1977) unqualified attack on left-wing influences in higher education, has been persuasive. It encouraged an interpretation of the process of schooling as being hijacked by progressives with their child-centred philosophies, open plan learning environments and mixed ability, multicultural objectives. These three dynamics were criticized as destroying the fabric of established practices, effective management and school discipline. With excellence sacrificed for mediocrity and directed learning strategies replaced by pupil choice, the child's potential – as an individual – was assumed to have been lost to the collective. As with other portrayals of 'childhood' in 'crisis', the reactionary backlash hankered after the golden age of its own childhood, when children knew their place, sat silent in rows, learned by rote the rudiments of the 3 Rs and were governed by harsh words and physical punishment.

As a result of government policy since the 1970s, a whole range of schools, from nursery through to sixth form, have borne the brunt of swingeing budgetary cuts, dilapidated buildings, overcrowded classrooms, out-of-date equipment and poor essential resources. Every local authority has its hierarchy of schools and the extension of parental choice, with finance tied to enrolment, has created the concept of the 'sink school'. The stress on teachers, and headteachers as managers, has been exacerbated by devolved and restricted budgets. While politicians and employers bemoan the lack of correspondence between school-based knowledge and skills and those demanded by industry, the reality for many young people, their families and communities is the lack of employment opportunity. The review of the welfare benefits system, virtually denying income support to 16- to 18-year-olds, has added to the frustration of an already demoralized youth. It is a demoralization restricted not only to the 'sink' schools of the inner cities and decaying towns. It extends throughout all schools and into further and higher education.

For over 20 years, critical educational theory, research, television documentaries and film drama, particularly the work of David Leland, have demonstrated that while private schools, grant maintained, and former grammar schools masquerading as comprehensives, have escaped virtually unscathed from chronic under-resourcing, there is a crisis in legitimacy throughout public sector education. Although structural inequalities inherent within postwar Britain prevailed throughout schooling – the private/state divide; the tripartite system of secondary state education; social class, gender and 'race' divisions – there was some recognition of social mobility aligned with meritocracy. However, much of the schooling process, from infant education through to school leaving, assisted in the reinforcement and maintenance of those structural inequalities. With restricted opportunities for upward social mobility, promoted by claims of opportunities-for-all, it soon became apparent that schools corresponded to the labour market and the needs of industry. But they decreasingly corresponded to the lives, experiences and aspirations of the children and young people on their rolls. Once structural unemployment became an institutionalized feature of contemporary society, the promise of trading hard work and commitment at school for a rewarding and secure future in the workplace became unrealizable. Effectively, for many young people, schools lost their relevance.

The question of the relationship between the role of schools and adulthood cannot be restricted to the confines of paid work opportunities, domestic responsibilities and social roles. It must be extended to include a commitment to a lifetime learning process; enabling children, young people and adults to realize their potentials, becoming informed and active citizens in an international context. This tension, between 'education' and 'schooling', has a long history and has been manifested over time in educational policy and legislation.

Schools for All

The arrival of mass education in Britain, through which all children attended school for much of their childhood, is often represented as a profound libertarian shift within society. Through schooling outside the home not only would children become literate, numerate and knowledgeable but also they would evolve as participants, as citizens-in-the-making. Schools were portrayed as sites of learning and preparation for future employment, roles and status. A persistent theme is that social change can be achieved through the personal development afforded within the formal processes of education. A century on from the advent of mass schooling, however, Eggleston argues that, far from releasing the intellectual and personal potential of its future citizens, schools and their curriculum transmit and legitimate knowledge and therefore 'become instruments of social control', helping to ensure 'the maintenance of the social system – its knowledge, its status, stratification and above all its power' (1977:3). While publicly adhering to the principle of inclusivity – educational opportunity for all – schools as institutions, both comparatively and internally, operate regimes based on exclusivity. Rather than being a vehicle for effectively challenging structural inequalities and social/cultural division, schools have assisted in their maintenance and reproduction.

Correspondence between school and work has a well-established history. Yet it was tied, through the late eighteenth century consolidation of 'education for all', to a broader shift in state intervention which involved all social institutions in the process of surveillance and regulation. As Baines acknowledged in 1846, 'A system of state education is a vast intellectual police force, set out to watch over the young', which prevents 'the intrusion of dangerous thoughts' and turns their minds 'into safe channels' (in Eggleston, 1977:32). Education was committed to 'gentling the masses' and, as Young and Whitty argue, schooling for the working classes 'could be as much a process of domestication as of liberation' (1977:1).

Essential to the development of educational priorities or objectives was the broader commitment to economic competitiveness and viability in developing world markets. Writing in 1868, Shuttleworth argued that 'more thorough primary instruction' and opportunities for 'superior education which leads to a knowledge of the technical relations of science and the arts' provided 'advantages' to 'foreign workmen'. Two years later, Foster argued that 'industrial prosperity' required 'speedy provision of elementary education' which would 'make up the smallness of our numbers by increasing the intellectual force of the individual' (in Wardle, 1974:53–4). A formalized commitment to the 'schooled child' and 'education for all' was conceptualized and expanded with successive increases in the minimum school leaving age (10 years in 1880; 11 years in 1893; 12 years in 1899; 14 years in 1918). Despite expansionist policies, educational opportunities remained dominated by gender and class inequalities. Yet the 1904 Elementary Code carried a commitment to forming and strengthening the character and the development of children's intelligence through public elementary schooling. Both girls and boys would be prepared 'according to their different needs . . . practically as well as intellectually, for the work of life'. Elementary schools were to train children in 'habits of observation and clear reasoning', acquaint them with the 'facts and laws of nature', familiarize them with the country's literature and history, give them 'some power over language as an instrument of thought and expression', and develop 'good reading' and 'thoughtful study'. The 'natural activities of hand and eye' were to be encouraged by 'practical work and manual instruction'. Health education, social development and sound discipline would 'implant in the children habits of industry, self-control ... perseverance ... a strong respect for duty ... and ... for others'. The Code emphasized the school as a community based on 'fair play' and 'loyalty', encouraging parental support and producing 'upright and useful members of the community in which they live, and worthy sons and daughters of the country to which they belong' (in Maclure, 1969:154–5).

The Regulations for Secondary Schools were also introduced in 1904, establishing the principle that such schools were of different types to meet the contrasting 'requirements of the scholars' and their 'place in the social organisation' as well as their future occupations and the demands of economic development. In 1906, Webb questioned how an efficient army could be formed from the 'stunted, anaemic, demoralized denizens of the slum tenements of our great cities', arguing that 'It is in the classrooms ... that the future battles of the Empire for commercial prosperity are already being lost' (in Wardle, 1974:54). The consolidation of the British Empire and international economic prosperity were key themes underpinning mass education and its attendant legislation. Early twentieth century education policy incorporated psychological, psychiatric and medical discourses supported by specialists in those fields. Much of their work centred on the assumed relationship between the physiological and the psychological development of children. The first Hadow Report noted the significance of the eleventh year in a child's development as 'presenting distinctive problems' which required a 'fresh departure in educational methods and organisation' (Board of Education, 1926:72). Further, for those children – the majority – not selected for Grammar schools, Hadow proposed the introduction of 'Modern' secondary schools geared to 'practical work and realistic studies' (Board of Education, 1926:xxiii). Within a colourful rhetoric of personal opportunity, fulfilment and growth, Hadow stressed the development of 'practical intelligence' towards 'the better and more skilled service of the community in all its multiple business and complex affairs'. The Report stressed the need for curriculum subjects to be practical, directly related to everyday life and connected to 'the interests arising from the social and industrial environment of the pupils' (Board of Education, 1926:176). This included gender 'appropriate' schooling so that girls could 'undertake intelligently the various household duties which devolve on most women' (Board of Education, 1926:234) and could be prepared for paid employment in the areas of dressmaking, millinery and needlecraft.

The primary–secondary school split at 11 years was affirmed in the second Hadow Report on primary education, which emphasized the significance of teaching based on interest and relevance for children of this age rather than requirements for later educational stages. To that end, Hadow argued that primary education should be experiential and activity-based; appealing 'more to the sympathy, social spirit and imagination of the children' than to 'passive obedience' and 'mass instruction', and encouraging the integration of 'individual and group work' (Board of Education, 1931:xvii–xviii). The philosophy of giving 7 to 11 year olds 'what is essential to their healthy growth – physical, intellectual and moral – during that particular stage of their development' (Board of Education, 1931:92) was extended to the third Hadow Report (Board of Education, 1933). This advocated infant and nursery provision based on child-centred play and discovery. Taken together, these proposals represented a significant shift towards the personal, social and cultural contexts of children although, at secondary level, the correspondence between school and work, be it paid or unpaid, in the jobs market or in the home, was now an established priority.

Given that secondary education was to correspond to the demands of the labour market and that it was a differentiated, class-based labour market, curriculum provision accordingly was also differentiated. A range of work of questionable methodology, geared to the measurement and predisposition of intelligence, had emerged from within the eugenics movement. When the Spens Report was published (Board of Education, 1938:357), psychologists were confident that, at a very early age, a child's 'innate all-round intellectual ability' could be tested and reliably predicted. The Report concluded that 'if justice is to be done to their varying capacities' (Board of Education, 1938:358) children from the age of 11 should receive differentiated education. Significantly, the Report noted that there was 'no clear line of demarcation, physical, psychological or social' between children at Grammar and those at Modern schools. Evidence about methods of selection confirmed their opinion that 'the line as drawn at present is always artificial and often mistaken' (Board of Education, 1938:140). It proposed the introduction of 'Technical' schools to establish a tripartite system of Grammar, Technical and Modern secondary education. The Norwood Report, however, noted the quite different outcomes resulting from each type of school. Grammar schools corresponded to the 'learned professions' (Board of Education, 1943:2) and management posts while Technical schools were craft-oriented in their applied curricula and Modern schools were concerned to provide for children who dealt 'more easily with concrete things than with ideas' (Board of Education, 1943:3). Norwood advocated continuation of this system but recommended easy transfer from one type of school to another as 'differentiation at 10 or 11+ cannot be regarded as final' (Board of Education, 1943:17). By the mid-1940s, schooling for all had been achieved and many of the progressive principles of education, often thought to have come later, were already in place. But so too was the hierarchical structure of British education, reflecting and reinforcing established inequalities, corresponding and sensitive to the demands of a developing monopoly capitalist economic system.

This is not to argue that there has been no social mobility within society. There has, particularly in the period of economic reconstruction post-1945, and schools have played a not insignificant part in this process. Educational opportunity, however, has remained closely associated with economic, particularly industrial, demands. There is clearly a tension between education as an end-in-itself and schooling for jobs, for industry. It is often manifested as a tension between intellectual endeavour and applied skills. Whatever the dynamics of this debate within educational theory, the postwar emphasis within education was that of correspondence between schools as places of preparation, and employment as the place of production.

Schooling the Meritocracy

The 1943 White Paper on Educational Reconstruction, the precursor to the 1944 Education Act, set the agenda for long-term educational reform in the context of 'the general picture of social reconstruction' (Board of Education, 1943b:4). A 'happier childhood', a 'better start in life' and a 'fuller measure of education and opportunity' were the priorities for children (Board of Education, 1943b:3). The intention was 'to provide means for all of developing the various talents with which they are endowed and so enriching the inheritance of the country whose citizens they are.' A policy balance was to be struck between 'diversity' and 'equality of educational opportunity'. As with late eighteenth century reforms, however, the explicit aim was to establish an 'educational system which will open the way to a more closely knit society' (Board of Education, 1943b:3). It was clear that those returning from war, and those who had suffered privation and tragedy at home, would not accept a long-term return to the deep depression of the 1930s. Education reform, along with Beveridge's 'war on poverty' and the establishment of the National Health Service, was part of a new, optimistic era of state intervention directed towards economic reconstruction and welfare provision.

In this context, of Keynesian economics and emerging socialism, a 'national education service' (Board of Education, 1943b:3) was envisaged – providing continuous schooling from nurseries, which had been so significant as part of the war effort, through to school leaving extended to 15 years (with 16 as the eventual objective). Reduction in primary school class sizes, improved accommodation and facilities, and secondary education 'of diversified types but of equal standing' (Board of Education, 1943b:3), were named priorities. The White Paper condemned selection at 11 and the negative impact of a 'cramped and distorted curriculum' (Board of Education, 1943b:6) which over-emphasized examinations and fostered competitiveness while stifling curiosity and imagination. The privileged position of Grammar schools was questioned and demands made for equivalence in resources and opportunities throughout secondary education. The 1944 Education Act changed the role of the state from that of supervision to one of intervention. Responsibility for the education of the people of England and Wales was placed at the door of the Minister of Education. Local Education Authorities (LEAs) were required to carry out their duties under the control and direction of this Minister. Development of technical education (1945 Percy Report) and University expansion (1946 Barlow Report) remained priorities to service industrial expansion and capital reconstruction.

Despite the overt commitment to equality of educational opportunity, schooling remained dogged by its structural, hierarchical divisions. Public schools remained untouched by state educational reform, with the wealthy retaining direct access to the privileges of private education from preparatory schools through to prestigious university education. The Early Leaving Report (Central Advisory Council for Education, 1954) showed conclusively that, within the state sector, access to Grammar schools and to certificated educational achievement was closely related to the occupations of fathers, concluding 'we do not assume that this is solely due to environment.' Rather than challenging the class-based system of stratified educational opportunity, however, the significance of increasing social mobility within it was emphasized. The foundations were laid upon which a meritocratic society could be achieved – through social mobility aided and abetted by educational achievement. The objective was to enable more children from non-professional backgrounds to become 'successful' within state education.

Although there were increased opportunities for the majority of children from working-class backgrounds, due to the expansionism of capital reconstruction and the ever-growing public sector, their 'success' was achieved despite the system rather than because of it (Reid, 1978). Nowhere was this more apparent than in the struggles of established black and Irish communities, and the expanding African Caribbean immigrant communities. English monoculturalism was serviced by educational policy and practice. At all levels of curriculum delivery, the experiences of working class and 'ethnic' communities were denied legitimacy. An emphasis on 'integration' was a metaphor for assimilation, and there was no recognition of the importance or value of cultural diversity. Similarly, the gender-differentiations of pre-war society, despite the role reversals of the war effort, were reaffirmed. Academic theorists such as Bowlby (1953) were enlisted to substantiate government-supported initiatives to return women to the home; their primary roles as wives, mothers, carers and domestic labourers secured for the 'good of the nation'. The 'woman behind the man behind the gun' became the 'woman behind the man behind the job'.

The correspondence between schooling, industry and economic expansion remained a central concern, with the 1956 White Paper on Technical Education seeking to 'strengthen the foundations of our economy', improve living standards and 'discharge effectively our manifold responsibilities overseas'. This would be achieved through increased industrial output, productive investment, high quality exports and competitively priced goods and services – underpinned by advances in technical education. The main purpose of such education was teaching pupils to be adaptable, although it was stressed that 'a place must always be found in technical education for liberal education' to ensure a broad outlook. The Paper concluded 'we cannot afford either to fall behind in technical accomplishments or to neglect spiritual and human values' (in Maclure, 1969:239–41). The Crowther Report on the education of 15- to

18-year-olds also argued against a narrow concentration on the 'immediate vocational target', rejecting much college education as 'mere instruction' (Central Advisory Council for Education, 1959:369). It criticized congestion of the curriculum in the final two years of secondary education and over-specialization at sixth form leading to limited content and choice. It also endorsed the 'principle of specialisation, or intensive study' (Central Advisory Council for Education, 1959:261), while recommending that the sixth form curriculum should include elements 'to develop the literacy of science specialists and the numeracy of arts specialists' (Central Advisory Council for Education, 1959:269).

The Crowther Report considered the physical, emotional and social development of young people. It recommended the raising of the school leaving age to 16 since 15-year-olds were thought 'not sufficiently mature to be exposed to the pressures of the world of industry or commerce' (Central Advisory Council for Education, 1959:108). Yet it proposed the consolidation of gender differentiation – stating: 'There can be no doubt that at this stage boys' thoughts turn most often to a career, and only secondly to marriage and the family' while 'the converse obtains with girls.' Thus 'sound educational policy' should 'take account of natural interests' – offering a 'curriculum which respects the different roles they play' (Central Advisory Council for Education, 1959:34). Such differentiation was reinforced by the Newsom Report which stated that 'for all . . . girls there is a group of interests relating to what many, perhaps most of them, would regard as their most important vocational concern, marriage' (Central Advisory Council for Education, 1963:37). Newsom focused on 13- to 16-year-olds of 'average' or less than average ability, recognizing that the kind of intelligence measured by tests was largely acquired, rather than genetic, and was influenced considerably by the social and physical environments of individuals. This led to 'much unrealized talent especially among boys and girls whose potential is masked by inadequate powers of speech and the limitations of home background' (Central Advisory Council for Education, 1963:3). Concern was expressed in the Report over 'slum' schools, poverty, poor health and 'delinquency' – to be remedied by compensatory programmes and school-based social work.

The Newsom Report reinforced previous assumptions about the nature of educational provision and the inducement for reform was 'the economic argument for investing in our pupils'. Future employment patterns would require 'a much larger pool of talent' and 'a generally better educated and intelligently adaptable labour force' (Central Advisory Council for Education, 1963:5). The 1963 Industrial Training Bill echoed this theme, maintaining that an increase in industrial skills training would secure steadier and more rapid economic growth. The Robbins Report on higher education reflected the importance of social restraints on wider educational opportunity, arguing an expansionist case on the basis that a 'highly educated population is essential to meet competitive pressures in the modern world'. It noted 'large reservoirs of untapped ability . . . especially among girls' and proposed an expansion of higher education to respond to demand (Committee on Higher Education, 1963:268).

In 1965, LEAs were given 12 months to submit plans for the reorganization of secondary education through comprehensivization – in line with the government's intention to end selection at 11+ (Department of Education and Science, 1965). The move towards comprehensive education reflected deep concerns over the negative effects of selection and streaming in secondary schools. The Plowden Report (Department of Education and Science, 1967), considering primary education, noted three challenges to selection for secondary education: the 'accuracy' of the process; differential and unfair provision for children of differing ability; the effect of segregation on achievement. Its social divisiveness, reinforcing rather than challenging the prevailing class structure, was also noted. Within 20 years of the 1944 Education Act the tripartite system had failed to deliver a meritocratic process and, in fact, had consolidated privilege. Plowden provided a mass of documented evidence to demonstrate the institutionalization of inequalities through streaming, which was said to favour girls, older pupils and middle-class children who were over-represented in upper streams and assigned more experienced teachers, better classrooms and generous resources. The Report concluded that a 'happy school' and 'atmosphere conducive to learning' had more to do with teacher attitudes, good practice and respect for children as individuals than testing, streaming and selection (Department of Education and Science, 1967:291).

Once again the key principles of the 1931 and 1933 Hadow Reports were confirmed: primary schools should promote learning through experience, self-discovery, creative topic-based work and individual advancement within a flexible and positive environment. Plowden emphasized curiosity, interest and enjoyment, and a view of 'work' and 'play' as complementary rather than oppositional. It demanded the establishment of Educational Priority Areas (EPAs) to redress social and economic disadvantage through compensatory investment of staff and resources. The expansion of nursery education was again recommended, along with incentives for teachers to work in EPAs. While Plowden was criticized for its patronizing tone and assumptions that working class families were inadequate in providing children with opportunities for constructive play, stimulating conversation, extensive vocabularies and 'intellectual interests', it argued that communities within EPAs had a right to 'positive discrimination' which could 'only succeed if a larger share of the nation's resources is devoted to education' (Department of Education and Science, 1967:53).

As Young and Whitty argue, however, the problem that emerged was one of identifying 'correlations between cultural features of working-class life and failure at school – factors which then became "deficiencies" for which educational policy-makers attempted to devise programmes of compensation' (1977:4). The appeal of such policies was a combination of contemporary philanthropy, a more malleable labour force and a renewed 'gentling of the masses'. During the late 1960s and early 1970s, these policies were challenged by an emerging critique of schools – their authority, curricula, attainment criteria, correspondence and legitimacy (Berg, 1973; Bowles and Gintis, 1976; Dale, Esland and MacDonald, 1976; Evetts, 1973; Morrish, 1972; Musgrove, 1965; Tapper and Salter, 1978; Young, 1971). It was proposed that, while children undoubtedly could achieve through institutionalized schooling, it was an achievement via conformity and opportunity which remained tightly constrained and constraining. Language and communication were good examples of the potential of social rejection and exclusion simply because of dialect, vocabulary or 'restricted codes' (Bernstein, 1972). More critical views of education suggested that all children, all cultures and subcultures, all communities and all families were to be valued for their experiences, quality of life and rationality on their own terms (Barton and Meighan, 1978).

Part of a broader radical review was international debate around 'deschooling' (Freire, 1972; Goodman, 1971; Holt, 1973; Illich, 1971), underpinned by a range of 'alternative' projects including inner-city 'free schools' and a growing middle-class trend towards home tuition (see Shotton, 1993; Wright, 1989). Much of the radical debate shared common ground, particularly the concern that schools restricted, rather than stimulated, personal growth and development. As Wardle notes, the 'de-schoolers' identified schools as fundamentally conservative agencies, 'so indoctrinating their pupils that they fear radical change, or cannot even conceive of its possibility' and possessing 'an uncontrolled power of distributing life chances' (1974:viii).

The 'radical challenge' undoubtedly had some impact on mainstream education and by the early 1970s 'diversity', of class, ethnicity or culture, were part of the national debate (Cosin *et al.*, 1971, 1977; Dale *et al.*, 1981; Flude and Ahier, 1974; Lawton, 1977). Multiculturalism, although often confused and contradictory in its definitions, was promoted as essential to the development of positive self-image among 'ethnic groups' and tolerance or sympathetic understanding on the part of white people in Britain's multiracial communities. Within the curriculum, teaching about different cultures, acknowledging and valuing 'difference', was promoted. The 1973 Select Committee Report on Race Relations and Immigration proposed measures for increased communication with, and participation of, 'ethnic minority' parents, community members, teachers, child-care professionals and welfare assistants. The 1977 Select Committee on Race Relations and Immigration Report, and an earlier Community Relations Commission Report (1974), called for the monitoring and review of assessment of 'ethnic minority children' and statistics relating to those defined as ESN (educationally subnormal). The emphasis on 'cultural pluralism' continued into the 1980s (Schools Council, 1982; Swann Report, 1985).

While there was considerable discussion around sex discrimination, including legislation in 1975, the gendered curriculum and gender differentiation persisted throughout education. Increased investment in girls was determined by a utilitarian approach based on widening the pool of skilled labour for the jobs market. Both DES and DHSS White and Green Papers confirmed the role of schools in preparing pupils for 'parenthood' and gender appropriate, heterosexual behaviour in relationships. Apart from the political–economic imperatives governing paid and unpaid work, and domestic labour, the school was identified as a primary site for moral guidance and instruction (see Chapter 4). Curriculum option availability; teacher and parent expectations; curriculum content; staffing and resources – each contributed to the reinforcement of sex-stereotyped perceptions of 'gender-appropriate' roles and status.

For all the claims made concerning policy changes aimed at creating a more egalitarian education system – nursery provision; raising of the school leaving age; language enrichment programmes; compensatory initiatives; comprehensivization – the key structural inequalities in Britain remained evident within schools and their outcomes. Any upward social mobility that had occurred since 1945 was more the result of an expanding political economy and a burgeoning middle class than fundamental advances in equal educational opportunity. Just as opportunities had opened up for a relatively small number of working-class children in the 1960s, so they closed down in the late 1970s as Britain endured a series of economic recessions leading to the return of structural unemployment. Schools were not the sites of creativity, self-realization and liberation of the individual. They were defined and consolidated by the requirements of capital reconstruction. In this context equal opportunities had been more concerned with 'supporting existing economic principles and Liberal democratic politics than with addressing structural issues concerning power and its relations' (Coppock, Haydon and Richter, 1995:47).

Ironically, mainstream political discourse, particularly that of the New Right led by Shadow Education Minister Margaret Thatcher, attacked education policies and practices for failing children, parents and industry because of progressive ideology. The politicization of school 'deviance' (Barton and Meighan, 1979) also continued. Young and Whitty argue that the Right sought to protect its 'beloved themes of elitism, standards and tradition' through proposing a 'return to traditional standards of morality and excellence, an emphasis on didactic teaching and public accountability of schools and the preservation of selective and independent schools' (1977:4).

Thatcher's Children

The late 1960s and early 1970s was a period of increasing civil protest and industrial conflict in Western Europe and North America. International concerns over the Vietnam War and South African apartheid combined with issues around trade union, welfare and civil rights to produce a new wave of popular activism. Central to this development was a loose coalition of radical students committed to establishing a coherent student movement (Wright,

1989). They questioned and challenged the role of the state, particularly the international interests of western political economies, and the complicity of their universities and colleges in supporting oppressive state policies. What passed as education, delivered in school and higher education curricula alike, was contested as being determined by the political interests, as well as economic needs, of the advanced capitalist state. The 'student movement', while never extending to all campuses and touching only a few schools, was represented as a crisis in higher education indicative of a wider anti-authority shift within schools. These developments coincided not only with a critical questioning of the role and function of schooling in advanced capitalist economies, but also with the most severe economic downturn to hit postwar western political economies. The British economy was 'in decline' (Gamble, 1981) and western capitalism was 'in crisis' (Gamble and Walton, 1976; Hall *et al.*, 1978).

Ironically, schools were berated for failing to prepare young people for the transition to work. It was argued that school-leavers did not have the appropriate skills, attitudes or qualities necessary for employment. In 1976 James Callaghan initiated the Great Debate on education focusing on four key issues: a common curriculum; monitoring 'standards'; teacher training; the correspondence between school and work. The Green Paper, *Education in Schools: A Consultative Document* (DES 1977), recommended the involvement of industry and commerce in curriculum planning and a review of the potential of a core curriculum which could prepare young people for the transition to adult and working life. It suggested that schools should be accountable to governing bodies with policy decisions shared between teachers, LEAs, the local community and parents. The 'HMI model' of a flexible common curriculum, integrating a 'tempered, moderate, humanistic ... version of the three Rs with much room for student choice, teacher professionalism and considerable ... local autonomy' (Paquette, 1991:104), was reduced by the New Right to a narrower concept. As part of the 1979 Thatcherite agenda to 'return to Victorian values', a prescribed National Curriculum would be clearly, if not rigidly, defined to include a core of traditional subject disciplines. Didactic teaching of specific and approved knowledge would be underpinned by objectives, efficiency, examinations and results. Lawton (1994), in his close analysis of the speeches and publications of successive Conservative education ministers, demonstrates the considerable impact of New Right ideology on educational policy and practice (see Ball, 1990; Bowe, Ball and Gold, 1992; Chitty, 1989, 1992; Chitty and Simon, 1993).

As Secretary of State for Education (1981–6), Sir Keith Joseph used a rhetoric of 'choice', 'excellence' and school opportunities for all but retained an emphasis on 'differentiation', 'relevance', 'vocationalism' and 'fitness for purpose'. It was his intention that 'less able' pupils should receive basic practical education and training separate from secondary academic education. He introduced the Technical and Vocational Education Initiative (TVEI), located in and funded by the Department of Industry and designed to improve the status of technical and vocational work. For the 14–18-year-olds involved, the focus was 'education for capability'; relating the skills of investigation, problem-solving, design and group work to the 'real world' of work. Yet it was a world of seriously diminished work opportunities for school-leavers. The teaching of 'Life and Social Skills' or 'Coping Skills' to the young unemployed was promoted, although these overtly focused on conformity and were of little relevance to those who were disillusioned about their material future. In 1983 the Youth Training Scheme was a further initiative aimed at the 16–18-year-old working-class unemployed. They were offered £20 per week to attend a 12-month training programme, most of which was 'on the job', aimed at equipping them with 'transferable skills' and the 'discipline of work'. Employers often exploited the scheme as providing a supply of no-cost labour, and sex inequalities were strongly reinforced (Cockburn, 1987). Critics argued that the new vocational initiatives were intended primarily to produce docile workers to serve the new industrial revolution (Bates *et al.*, 1984). Young people themselves expressed feelings of being disenfranchised and perceived such schemes 'to be for keeping people off the street' (in Fiddy, 1984:170).

Having argued that teacher training institutions had become infected by progressive theories, thereby producing ineffective and inadequate teachers, Joseph set up the Council for the Accreditation of Teacher Education (CATE) in 1984. To be granted Qualified Teacher Status, teacher training courses had to be judged by HMI Inspectors who decided whether they met specific new criteria. The following year the Government published its Better Schools (DES, 1985) document, in which it argued that academic standards in schools were falling. Rather than taking note of HMI (1982) warnings concerning under-resourcing of schools, it targeted unplanned and ineffectively taught curriculum content; decontextualized teaching of basic literacy and numeracy skills; limited practical, scientific work; over-directive teaching; low teacher expectations. In short, children were failing, standards were falling, and teaching was to blame. The solution was to be found in the familiar areas of the curriculum; assessment as a means of monitoring 'standards'; teacher effectiveness and management of the profession; the governance of schools. With 'progressive' teaching, inappropriate curricula and lack of accountability identified as the roots of the 'crisis' in the classroom, the stage was set for further legislation to affirm New Right ideology.

As Education Minister (1986–9), Kenneth Baker extended the criticisms of progressive teaching to include what he identified as an 'in-house' ideology within the Department for Education and Science (DES). Civil servants were allegedly in league with teaching unions, education academics, teacher trainers and LEAs, and their egalitarian ideals, supposedly dominating schooling and inspection, were said to be anti-excellence, anti-selection and anti-market. Baker was committed to the competition of market forces, arguing that parental choice would be better served in such a climate. Standards would be increased through a broad, balanced curriculum, regular testing and publication of results. Selection, choice and diversity would be established through different types of status for schools and changes in budgetary control and school management. The enabling legislation soon followed. Under the 1986 Education (No 2) Act, school governing bodies were devolved responsibilities previously held by LEAs. These included the school curriculum; the monitoring and regulation of teaching of partisan political views; new systems of pupil exclusion; annual reports and parental consultation; sex education policies.

The 1988 Education Reform Act gave the Secretary of State for Education over 400 new powers. This centralization of operational powers was in contrast to the political rhetoric of the free market and devolution. In fact, as the shift in budgetary responsibility from LEAs to individual school governing bodies (Local Management of Schools: LMS) showed, the prime objective was to dissipate the powers of LEAs. Schools could now opt out of LEA control, gaining centrally-funded grant-maintained (GM) status. A policy of open enrolment was adopted ostensibly to provide parents with a wider choice of school provision. City Technology Colleges (CTCs) were set up to provide technical and vocational education for 11- to 19-year-olds in private institutions relying on government and private sector funding, although the latter has been less than forthcoming.

The 1988 Act established a National Curriculum for all maintained schools consisting of statutory content in nine subjects: English, Mathematics and Science (core); Technology, Geography, History, Physical Education, Art, Music (foundation). Compulsory testing was introduced through Standard Assessment Tasks (SATs) at 7, 11 and 14 years, and all children were required to attend daily an act of worship, unless withdrawn by parents. Attainment targets and programmes of study specified curriculum content, with general level descriptions or end of Key Stage statements outlining expected attainment for pupils aged 5 to 16 years. Following several revisions, the content remains knowledge-based, ethnocentric and reflective of New Right ideology. The only tacit acknowledgement of cultural diversity is in the Art and Music National Curriculum documents. Sex education in Key Stages 1 (5–7 years) and 2 (7–11 years) is limited to the narrowly defined Science curriculum – focusing on reproduction as one of the processes of life and the stages of the human life cycle. The 1993 Education Act transferred teaching about HIV, AIDS and sexually transmitted diseases from the Key Stage 3 (11–14 years) Science curriculum to Sex Education, from which parents can withdraw their children.

The compulsory National Curriculum was accompanied by non-statutory documentation from the now disbanded National Curriculum Council (NCC). The NCC recommended the fostering of 'a climate in which equality of opportunity is supported by a policy to which the whole school subscribes and in which the positive attitudes to gender equality, cultural diversity and special needs of all kinds are actually promoted' (1990:3). Such important objectives, however, have been overshadowed by a climate of testing and assessment of attainment as providing information on individual performance within a standardized, national framework. Questioning of the relevance and purpose of blanket testing, and publication of results in league tables, was sufficient to bring disclosure of the Conservative Government's thinking. In 1991 Kenneth Clarke, Education Secretary (1990–2), argued, 'The British Left believe that pencil and paper examinations impose stress on pupils and demotivate them . . . This remarkable national obsession lies behind the more vehement opposition . . . to 7-year-old testing.' He claimed, 'This opposition to testing and examinations is largely based on a folk memory on the Left about the old debate on the 11+ and grammar schools' (in Lawton, 1994:99–100). Despite well organized and persistent resistance by parents, teachers, educationalists and the unions, the tests on 7-, 11- and 14-year-old children have become little more than formal, pencil and paper exercises in the core subjects. The 1992 Schools Act formalized publication of league tables showing examination results and attendance levels in secondary schools, and annual reports for all pupils. Reports for 7-, 11- and 14-year-olds also provide individual levels of attainment and comparisons with peers/national averages in core subjects. The stated intention was to produce standardized test results as a 'measure of standards', promoting 'parental choice' through 'reliable' indicators of 'good' or 'poor' schools while increasing the accountability of teachers, headteachers and governing bodies. In 1996 Gillian Shephard, Secretary of State for Education, reversed the decision that primary schools should not publish SAT results in league tables, arguing that revelation of results will help improve standards in numeracy and literacy. Fierce resistance has resulted in the National Association of Headteachers encouraging governing bodies to refuse publication – thus breaking the law by not fulfilling a statutory duty. The 1992 Act also established the Office for Standards in Education (OFSTED). The latter comprises privatized inspection teams, which include non-educationalists, competing for inspection contracts enabling them to inspect schools every four years. Resulting reports, supposedly identifying strengths and weaknesses, recommending improvements and increasing accountability, are in the public domain. The 1993 Education Act gave powers to the Education Secretary to establish associations to run any school judged by OFSTED to have low standards or regarded as failing and close the school if this does not lead to change.

Kenneth Clarke advocated National Vocational Qualifications (NVQs), to be on a par with the narrow curriculum contained in the 'A' levels taught to a minority of 16–18-year-olds. He actively supported a curriculum of categorized subjects emphasizing knowledge and British cultural heritage. He attacked left-wing, progressive views of expert educationalists, and maintained that comprehensive education is an obstacle to democratic society. In 1992 he announced the reform of teacher training and plans for less education theory, more school-based practice, and use of 'mentor' teachers in schools working in 'partnership' with training institutions. Statements of competence would be introduced to provide a framework for, and evaluate, course effectiveness. At the 1992 Conservative Party Conference the Prime Minister, John Major, revealed the underlying ideological position in his plea for a 'return to basic subject teaching, not courses in the theory of education' (in Lawton, 1994:74). He argued that primary teachers 'should learn how to teach children to read', implying that this did not happen, 'not waste their time on the politics of gender, race and class' (1994:74).

The imposition of centralized control throughout the 1980s extended to further and higher education with the autonomy of universities also reduced by the 1988 Education Reform Act, making them directly accountable to the Secretary of State for Education. The University Grants Council was replaced by the Higher Education Funding Council (HEFC) with members from industry and commerce appointed by the Education Secretary. Many former polytechnics and colleges gained university status, no longer to be the responsibility of local authorities. Given the contemporary shift to market-led, cost-efficient higher education under a central funding agency, it is worth noting a statement by the Chair of the 1945 Percy Report, stating government policy of that time was 'based on the principle that a university should be a self-governing community of teachers and students, working together in one place, mature enough to set its own standards of teaching and strong enough to resist outside pressures, public or private, political or economic' (in Maclure, 1969:229). 'Outside pressures' have been exerted on teacher training through the 1993 Education Bill (Teacher Education) which removed funding for teacher education from HEFC to the newly developed quango, the Teacher Training Agency (TTA). Its brief covers funding for initial teacher education, in-service education including higher degrees and educational research.

'Crisis' Revisited

A 1996 EU survey found that 'contrary to the Government's claims, Britain spends a lower percentage of its national wealth on education than any other European state', while 'British teachers take some of the biggest classes in some of the biggest schools in Europe, and for more hours than virtually anywhere else' (*Guardian*, 8 May 1996). Since 1980 the impact of legislative and policy change on education, from pre-school through to universities, has been profound. The threads running through educational reform, as identified above, represent the consolidation of the political ideology of the New Right. Increased central control, particularly the Education Reform Act (1988), significantly affected the former partnership relationship between the government, LEAs and schools in educational policy making (Bash and Coulby, 1989; Department of Cultural Studies, 1991; Maclure, 1992; McNay and Ozga, 1985). Critics, including those directly involved in policy initiatives, have warned of a government which refuses to listen to, and insulates itself from, professional opinion and expertise while enforcing politicized central control which is often based on ministerial opinion (see Chitty and Simon, 1993). While each education minister has promoted personal priorities, the broader context has remained consistent. The role of schools in the social and physical development of pupils has been undermined as, for example, the requirement for LEAs to provide school meals (except for children whose families receive state benefits) was removed and nursery provision was made discretionary under the 1980 Education Act. The commitment within the curriculum has been to 'core' subjects, with content and assessment imposed nationally to guarantee conformity and restrict exploration and diversity within the learning process. Both the National Curriculum and other, vocationally-oriented initiatives, have reaffirmed the correspondence between school and work (Ainley, 1988; Corson, 1991; Hollands, 1991). The renaming of the Department for Education *and Employment* (DFEE) reinforces this relationship. The potential for other important objectives (health, sex and sexuality, citizenship, parenting) has been severely limited if not actively discouraged. Lawton argues strongly that 'a potentially modernising curriculum reform was predictably bungled by a mixture of incompetence, reactionary prejudice and suspicion' (1994:136–7). Its emphasis on discrete subjects and traditional testing, together with the judgmental style of monitoring and inspection, reflect an implicit distrust of teachers' professional judgement. The political rhetoric accompanying successive education reforms has encouraged a persistent media-hyped attack on teaching standards and academic quality.

Conceptually, the process of schooling has been returned to structures derived in hierarchical assumptions about intelligence, ability and, inevitably, selection. 'Child-centred', 'holistic', 'experiential' and 'responsive' classroom approaches have been vilified as being the substance of a contemporary progressivism which has left the nation bereft of literate, numerate and motivated young people. Chris Woodhead, Chief Inspector of Schools, has affirmed these assertions. However, considerable concern has been expressed within OFSTED about the basis of such claims, and 'the evidence on which the Chief Inspector makes his pronouncements is increasingly being called into question' as 'inspectors talk . . . of "doctoring", "slanting", even "distortion"' (*Observer*, 5 May 1996). Despite such criticisms, the New Right has maintained that a return to 'basics', by which it means the didactic delivery of skills and facts within a competitive market-place of schooling in which regular assessment becomes the public measure of a school's success, will bring the best from teachers and pupils. If governors and headteachers are forced to compete for resources, including funds related to enrolment, the assumption is that schools as mini-businesses will thrive.

The reintroduction of selection, however, has emphasized social divisions that postwar schooling, including comprehensivization, never managed to eradicate. Open enrolment has led to popular schools selecting their intake, thus exacerbating the problems faced by so-called 'sink' schools since the consequent decline in their numbers necessarily results in reduced finance. This, in turn, affects staffing ratios, maintenance of buildings, resourcing, etc. Middle-class children, with the added material benefits of professional and relatively well-off parents who understand and use the system and can afford to transport their children to schools outside their locality, gain access to schools with better reputations. For children in poorer areas, the disadvantages of less favourable conditions and resources are a direct result of the choices made by others. At the same time, the decrease in financial resources of LEAs – brought about by the opting out of some schools – has had negative effects on those remaining under LEA control. Provision of services for preschool children, those with special needs or who do not speak English as their first language, have each been reduced while provision of facilities such as libraries, swimming instruction and tuition for music have been curtailed, if not removed.

Contrary to government claims, research by Ben and Chitty (1995) demonstrates that standards have consistently risen over the last 30 years, and that streaming pupils by ability does not guarantee better examination results or entry into higher education. Above average academic results and staying-on rates were recorded in comprehensives not competing with selective schools in the same area. However, those forced to compete with selective schools achieved below average performance – leading Ben and Chitty to conclude that government support for selectivity is the greatest threat to raising standards. The much proclaimed egalitarianism of comprehensive education has also been undermined particularly by material realities. The elite, private schools are massively resourced. Beneath these, well beyond the reach of most people, are opted out grant-maintained schools which have received disproportionately generous funding (Association of Metropolitan Authorities, 1993), and the partly privately-funded CTCs. At the base of the system are competing LEA schools. Research by the Child Poverty Action Group (Smith and Noble, 1995) concludes that education policy changes since 1979 have exacerbated barriers to learning and opportunities for the 'socially disadvantaged'. In those communities enduring the worst excesses of structural unemployment and a low income base, families are least able to provide material or personal support to their children and local schools. This widens the differential between those schools and others with middle-class intakes whose school trips, essential resources and necessary facilities are supplemented by professional wage-earners. In addition, subsidized places for 'academically able' working-class children in independent schools – via the assisted places scheme – and places in CTCs have generally not been offered to, or sought by, the parents of such children.

The 1988 Education Reform Act was premised on the notion of equality of opportunity for all pupils. As Troyna (1993:79) argues, however, 'that entitlement cannot be genuinely offered within an institutional and ideological framework which sanctions the maintenance, reproduction and extension of inequality.' While the National Curriculum gives the appearance of open access to core and foundation subjects for all school students up to the age of 14, falling school rolls and budgetary cuts have had a significant impact on resourcing which has seriously inhibited curriculum development in many schools. Beyond this, the 'hidden curriculum', through which low expectations, negative attitudes and harassment relating to gender, race, class, and ability have become institutionalized, has remained unchallenged by policy reforms. The interpersonal dynamics of the classroom and the playground have resulted in restricted opportunities, under-achievement and negative self-esteem for many pupils and students. As research since the late 1970s and early 1980s has illustrated, although structural relations constrain possibilities, they do not fully determine what occurs in schools. Classrooms are sites of negotiation concerning daily interaction between pupils, staff, pupils and staff (Delamont, 1976, 1983, 1984; Hammersley and Woods, 1984; Woods, 1979, 1980a, 1980b). Further, some pupils and teachers actively resist, challenge and reject what they consider to be inappropriate rules and regimes – either within schools (Griffin, 1985; Hudson, 1984; Lees, 1986; McEwan, 1991; McLaren, 1986; Walker and Barton, 1983; Wood, 1984) or by choosing to truant (Carlen, Gleeson and Wardhaugh, 1992). However, as Coppock *et al.* state, 'The National Curriculum is the ultimate exercise in liberal reformism as it proposes reform via curriculum content, organisation and resources but fails to deal with other power-related issues' (1995:72). In fact, the social, political and economic relations of structural inequality, exacerbated through high levels of unemployment and an ever-expanding poor, have been emphasized within schools rather than effectively challenged. There is little room for the principles of compensatory education in schools whose cost effectiveness and value-for-money is assessed in the market-place of competition, where the focus is on academic achievement and school attendance, and where notions of future 'citizenship' emphasize responsibility, discipline and conformity through control and regulation.

Under the 1988 Education Reform Act, the curriculum in schools should actively promote the 'spiritual, moral, cultural, mental and physical development of pupils' preparing them 'for the opportunities, responsibilities and experiences of adult life.' In principle such statements are laudable, implicitly recognizing diversity and providing a school experience accordingly. Yet, as discussed above, the radical right reformism of successive Conservative administrations has exacerbated rather than contested discrimination, both in policies and practices. Low priority has been given to establishing means of achieving and substantiating equality of opportunity and no statutory or policy framework has been introduced to promote anti-discriminatory curricula. The development of effective policies and strategies remains dependent on LEAs, individual schools, classroom teachers and the training received in teacher training institutions or through in-service courses. Even basic provision for essential language resources or non-Christian religious faiths is not necessarily available. These issues raise fundamental questions of statutory rights.

In the UK there is no recognition of the civil or political rights of the child in the process of schooling. The historical legacy of not listening to children in education continues (Davie and Galloway, 1996). With no guaranteed right of participation in decisions, children are expected to be passive observers of a process which identifies their parents or guardians as the 'consumers' of education. This extends to withdrawal from classes relating to health and welfare (sex education) and faith (religious education), and to special needs and exclusion proceedings. Education legislation incorporates no obligation to promote the rights of the child. The 'welfare principle', based on addressing the 'best interests of the child', does not extend to education provision and its administration. Issues of personal need are often subsumed under consideration of collective needs – of a class or school – when LEAs, governors, headteachers and staff take decisions regarding appropriate provision within a school. With no formal structure of complaints available, there is no access to clearly defined routes through which concerns can be raised and no recognition of children's rights to redress or grievance. Children are further marginalized from consultation or participation in decisions about school policy and administration, including matters such as the curriculum, uniform, meals, playground, discipline and extra-curricular activities. There is no provision for freedom of expression through dress, style, hair and often these issues lead to disciplinary action as schools invoke codes of conduct which were established without any consultation with pupils. Failure to comply with such rules regularly leads to suspension and, occasionally, to exclusion.

The imposition of the National Curriculum, with its detailed structure and specifically defined content, has inhibited teachers in their potential responses to the interests and needs of children, thus denying them freedom of expression. Connected with this has been the denial of children's rights to seek, receive and impart information and ideas, particularly concerning sex and sexuality education (see Chapter 4). Cuts in provision, and the introduction of charges for a range of tuition, have also limited freedom of expression through arts subjects. Corporal punishment has been abolished throughout maintained schools but this has not eradicated arbitrary uses of physical punishment or verbal abuse and humiliation by some teachers. Some schools, particularly special schools, use 'time out' rooms or cupboards to contain or punish 'difficult' children or those who persistently misbehave. Bullying in schools is also pervasive, particularly targeting children with special educational needs or those from ethnic communities. The Children's Rights Office has provided a systematic analysis of the extent to which UK law, its state policies and practices, comply with the UN Convention on the Rights of the Child (CRDU, 1994). This exposes a lack of commitment and adherence to even the most basic Articles.

After receiving and considering the UK's initial report, submitted four years after the ratification of the Convention, the UN Committee made a series of observations on the submission. While welcoming government initiatives concerning bullying, special educational needs and pre-school provision, it raised a number of concerns about 'matters relating to education'. These included: the right to appeal against school exclusions; the opportunity for children to express views on the running of schools; the familiarization of teachers with the UN Convention through training curricula incorporating education about the Convention; teaching methods inspired by and reflecting the spirit of the Convention; the introduction of education about the Convention into school curricula; the prohibition of corporal punishment in private schools. The Committee also proposed further support for integrated education and Irish language teaching in Northern Ireland, and 'proactive measures' for the rights of Gypsy and Traveller children, particularly their right to education.

The implementation of these recommendations depends on a realizable commitment to collective, cooperative work involving real partnerships between children and adults. This represents a challenge to the 'coincidence of interest' between adults which currently provides parents and guardians, teachers, headteachers, governors, education providers and politicians with the capacity to take decisions on behalf of children and young people without any requirement for consultation. In the debates over schools, colleges and universities, over curriculum content and school provision, over funding and the balance of resources, the voices of children and young people are rarely heard. Yet there is no shortage of opinion, discussion and direction emanating from adults who provide their, often ill-informed, constructions and interpretations of children's experiences, thoughts, knowledge and understanding. This adult version of childhood and schooling fails to identify the diversity and complexity of children's views, experiences and expectations, their language and conventions. It also systematically denies children access to essential information from which they can establish informed decisions about their lives.

In schools, children's participation should be formalized in the setting of policies, priorities and practices. There should be informed involvement in planning, monitoring and evaluating learning programmes and behaviour strategies. Classes should be consulted on the organization of the classroom, schemes of work and related activities – agreeing on working practices, expectations, rewards and sanctions. There is no justification for excluding pupils or students from school, college or university development plans, their associated policies and practices, or from review through regular consultation during informal discussion, in lessons and via School Councils. Within this developmental process of consultation, it is essential to establish curricula which are relevant to children, taking into account their life experiences and the impact of structural and social constraints on their lives. Curriculum content should be attentive to the individual as well as collective needs of children and young people, legitimating and building on their interests and skills rather than simply delivering content-laden subjects aimed at specific levels commensurate with specified ages. Cross-curricular skills, themes and dimensions should underpin school and higher education studies, and the hidden curriculum should be identified and acknowledged as a significant determinant of school life and its opportunities. In contrast to the narrow 'skills-for-work' approach of the last decades of the twentieth century, schools' pastoral systems and ethos should promote self-esteem and the education of the 'whole' child through objectives which do not necessarily deny the significance of achieved skills, required knowledge, or academic foundation in necessary subjects, but contextualize and position these within a broader educational framework.

At the heart of such developments, and reflective of the spirit of the UN Convention, inter-agency intervention in children's education must reflect the principle of the 'best interests of the child'. To this end, children and young people must be active participants in all decisions which affect their lives – with agencies working collectively rather than as single-issue, isolated professional bodies with limited agendas. It is essential that agencies cooperate and process specific issues or cases quickly, efficiently and fairly – thus reducing the potential for delays, inconsistencies and buck-passing. An emphasis on the 'protection' of children, and their perceived inability as informed decision-makers, together underpin current education and welfare responses. Professional practices are unlikely to change while academic theories and interventionist strategies continue to reinforce the structural and interpersonal vulnerabilities of children.

It is often assumed that children who do not attend school are 'uneducated', 'at risk', 'deviant' or 'criminal'. What has never been recognized within mainstream educational theory and practice is that schooling is but one area of childhood experiences and education. Compulsory schooling, for all its undeniable potential benefits, offers education within increasingly explicit and limited frameworks. These frameworks, now limited further by the imposition of a reactionary political agenda, have the capacity to reinforce and perpetuate oppression, prejudice, discrimination and inequalities at both attitudinal and institutional levels. Yet, schools can be liberative and classrooms can be the sites of realized potential. Schools are places in which relations of power can be challenged, where rights and responsibilities can be promoted, where the development of citizenship can occur over time, and where children can be encouraged to understand and exercise their rights as active participants.

Chapter 6

Children in Trouble: State Responses to Juvenile Crime

Barry Goldson

Juvenile Justice 1982–1992: A Fragile Consensus

Between 1982 and 1992 three principles underpinning statutory policy responses to children and young people in trouble emerged, developed and consolidated. Diversion, decriminalization and decarceration formed the cornerstones of an innovatory and unified approach comprising 'one of the most remarkably progressive periods of juvenile justice policy' (Rutherford, 1995:57). The formulation and application of these principles was directed and informed by a paradoxical coalescence between elements of academic research, professional practice developments in social work with juvenile offenders, specific policy objectives of Thatcherite Conservatism, and the stated imperatives of the police and the courts to protect the public and reduce the incidence of juvenile delinquency and anti-social behaviour. Each of these 'concerns' combined and formed a delicately balanced consensus guiding what became known as juvenile justice through the 1980s and into the 1990s (Goldson, 1994).

Academic research provided a consistent stream of empirical findings offering unequivocal evidence that for the vast majority of 'offending' children and young people, their anti-social behaviour was essentially petty and opportunistic and little more than a transitory phase that they would grow out of (Morris and Giller, 1983; Pitts, 1988; Pratt, 1985; Rutherford, 1986). Added to this was the work of the labelling theorists who focused on the impact of welfare and justice interventions in actually creating or sustaining delinquent behaviour. Blackmore notes:

> The labelling perspective is particularly relevant . . . as it focuses specifically on how the process of social control can affect delinquent behaviour. Traditionally the agencies of social control (police, schools, social services, probation and courts) were viewed as passive responders to delinquency. In other words they were seen as merely reacting to delinquent behaviour. However, labelling theorists have questioned this and instead focused attention on the ways that social control agencies react can in fact create and lead to further deviant behaviour (1984:45–6).

The message from the research was clear: premature and over-zealous interventions not only hindered the process of growing out of crime but also, by the application of criminal labels, could serve to compound the likelihood of further juvenile delinquency. Thus decriminalizing children's deviant behaviour and diverting them from formal welfare and justice interventions became principal objectives of juvenile justice policy and practice.

Further, research and inquiries, both independent and state funded, provided a wealth of compelling evidence indicating the futility and counter-productive nature of custodial responses to juvenile crime (Bottomley Committee, 1988; Thornton, 1984; Woolf Report, 1991). Such was the strength of this evidence that Pitts (1990:8) observes:

> In as much as social scientific research can ever 'prove' anything it has proved that locking up children and young people in an attempt to change their delinquent behaviour has been an expensive failure . . . more and more studies have demonstrated the tendency of these institutions to increase the reconviction rates of their ex-inmates, to evoke violence from previously non-violent people, to render ex-inmates virtually unemployable, to destroy family relationships and to put a potentially victimised citizenry at greater risk.

Apart from the issues raised by the imprisonment of children, in terms of conceptualizations of 'justice', 'welfare', and 'childhood' and concerns in relation to ethics and humanity, the research indicated that it had been a miserable and expensive failure when judged in terms of its own claims to deter and rehabilitate juvenile delinquents. It was this message that had a profound effect in establishing and prioritizing decarceration within juvenile justice.

Indeed, the principles of diversion, decriminalization and decarceration provided a solid foundation for professional social work practice with children and young people in trouble. Informed by the academics, a new orthodoxy and a powerful, progressive and confident mood shaped juvenile justice social work practice. The new justice oriented social work practice was galvanized further by the developing critique of spurious 'welfarist' notions of 'needology' and 'preventive' interventions with children considered to be at risk of offending, which had informed social work practice with children in trouble during the 1970s (Pratt, 1987; Thorpe *et al.*, 1980). A dynamic new practice developed and was underpinned by the principles of minimum necessary intervention, systems intervention, effective monitoring and campaigning, intra- and inter-agency networking, strategic diversionary approaches, and the provision of community supervision, specified activities and alternatives to custody (Allen, 1991; Pitts, 1990; Rutherford, 1992).

The positive interrelation between research and practice during this period developed within the space permitted by its paradoxical compatibility with discrete Thatcherite policy imperatives. Throughout the 1980s the Conservative Party was committed to relieving the Treasury of its public spending responsibilities and was determined to make swingeing cuts. As Pratt observes 'to reduce the custodial population on the grounds of cost effectiveness . . . led to a general support for alternatives to custody initiatives' (1987:429). Prominent MPs and Conservative ministers were keen to support the diversionary and decarcerative juvenile justice priorities with John Patten and Virginia Bottomley (in The Children's Society, 1993:17–18) in complete agreement:

> I think there is now a fairly wide consensus about what the response to juvenile offending should be . . . formal intervention should be kept to a minimum, consistent with the circumstances and seriousness of each case (John Patten, 18 March 1988).

> If anything, I have become firmer in my belief that penal custody remains a profoundly unsatisfactory outcome for children (Virginia Bottomley, 18 March 1988).

Indeed, during this period the legislative framework concerning criminal law experienced consistent and incremental progression, providing even greater space within which new juvenile justice policy and practice was able to develop. The 1982 Criminal Justice Act for the first time introduced a statutory basis for the provision of Social Inquiry Reports, tightened the criteria for imposing custodial sentences on juveniles and, through Section 20, provided for the Specified Activities Order whereby a programme of community-based activities might be specified to the court as an alternative to the imposition of custody. In 1983 the DHSS Local Authority Circular (LAC 83/3) facilitated the release of 15 million pounds to establish and develop alternative to custody projects for juveniles. This involved partnerships between national child-care non-statutory organizations and local authorities. In 1988 the government developed its juvenile justice thinking further through the publication of the Green Paper, *Punishment, Custody and the Community* (Home Office, 1988), in which it declared:

> most young offenders grow out of crime as they become more mature and responsible. They need encouragement and help to become law-abiding. Even a short period of custody is quite likely to confirm them as criminals, particularly as they acquire new criminal skills from more sophisticated offenders. They see themselves labelled as criminals and behave accordingly (1988: paras. 2.17–2.19).

The principles around which the Green Paper was shaped exuded the concepts and even adopted the very language of the academics and juvenile justice practitioners ('grow out of crime'; 'labelled'). Moreover, the Government was apparently so convinced with the merits of diversion, decriminalization and decarceration that it was its stated intention to further extend the use of cautioning and the range of community-based disposals in order to impose additional limits on custodial sentencing. Similarly, juvenile justice practice had been so successful that it would be extended to young adults as it was,

> particularly suitable for young men and women, who are likely to grow out of crime . . . The Government's proposals include:
> – less use of custody, particularly for thieves and burglars;
> – a new order, giving the courts powers to place a wide range of requirements on offenders who would now be given custodial sentences . . . (Home Office, 1988: paras. 2.17–2.19).

The 1988 Criminal Justice Act further tightened the criteria for custodial sentencing, and the 1989 Children Act abolished the Criminal Care Order as provided by Section 7(7) of the 1969 Children and Young Persons Act, placing instead a responsibility on local authorities to 'take reasonable steps designed to reduce the need to bring criminal proceedings against children' (1989 Children Act Schedule 2, Paragraph 7). Finally, the 1991 Criminal Justice Act consolidated the decarcerative priorities in relation to juvenile justice which had developed throughout the 1980s offering, via the establishment of the Youth Court, the potential to include 17-year-olds within its practice remit. Further, the 1991 Act abolished the use of prison custody for 14-year-old boys, provided for the abolition of prison remands for 15- and 16-year-olds (although this is still to be implemented), emphasized community sentences, and placed a duty on all engaged in the criminal justice process 'to avoid discriminating against persons on the grounds of race or sex or any other improper ground' (Section 95(1)(b)). This was the first time that such a provision had appeared in criminal law and implicitly it represented an acknowledgement of the institutionalized injustices of the justice process together with a commitment to remove them.

It is a curious paradox of the 1980s and early 1990s, a period in which occurred the most consistent, vitriolic and vindictive affronts to justice and welfare, that the legal framework provided the space within which the principles of diversion, decriminalization and decarceration in policy and practice with children in trouble became ascendant. Ostensibly the period was underpinned by a delicately balanced consensus, the final element of which included the police and the courts. While examples could be found where the courts and the police positively embraced the new principles of juvenile justice (Gibson, 1995:64), profound reservations and concerns remained. Nevertheless, it became increasingly difficult to sustain resistance in the face of the developing evidence and 'the scepticism, if not overt opposition, that existed within the police and the courts to the principles of diversion, decriminalisation and decarceration, was at least partially pacified by the plethora of Home Office research . . . that evidenced the discernible success of such policies' (Goldson, 1994:5). Repeated government guidance (Home Office Circular 14, 1985 and Home Office Circular 59, 1990) promoted diversionary strategies which resulted in a dramatic increase in the use of cautioning; by 1990, 70 per cent of boys and 86 per cent of girls aged between 14 years and 16 years who offended were cautioned by the police (Home Office, 1991). Similarly, the decarcerative 'juvenile justice' priorities produced a striking decrease in the use of custodial sentences for juveniles which fell from 7,900 in 1981 to 1,700 in 1990 (Home Office, 1991). However, most compelling was the apparent success of the new policy and practice direction, with the increased emphasis on diversion and decarceration producing a corresponding decrease in the incidence of juvenile delinquency. The Children's Society Advisory Committee observes:

> Home Office statistics suggest that there has been a 37 per cent decline in the number of known juvenile offenders since 1985. This is partly attributable to demographic changes – the juvenile population has fallen by 25 per cent. However, the number of known juvenile offenders per 100,000 of the population has also fallen, from 3,130 in 1980 to 2,616 in 1990, a drop of 16 per cent. It remains true that juveniles commit a high proportion of all detected offences but this also appears to be declining. In 1980 juvenile crime represented 32 per cent of all crime; in 1991 that figure has dropped to 20 per cent (1993:21).

It would be misleading to describe the developments in juvenile justice between 1982 and 1992 in terms of unqualified success; not least because the 'justice' which prevailed was permeated with institutional injustices. Although the impact of social class upon the processing of children and young people in trouble was making an increasing impression upon professional consciousness and practice (Box, 1981; Pitts, 1988), the more insidious influence of 'race' and gender determinants was essentially left unchecked. Indeed, the juvenile justice process was rife with attitudinal and institutional racism and sexism and, with some notable exceptions (for example, Mountain, 1988; National Intermediate Treatment Federation, 1986), even the 'progressive' practitioners tended to adopt 'colour blind' and 'gender blind' approaches. Black children and young people experienced racism at every point of the juvenile justice process (Commission for Racial Equality, 1992; Gilroy, 1987; Gordon, 1983) and more specifically during arrest and at the police station (Landau *et al.*, 1983; Scraton, 1982, 1985; Willis, 1983); in the courts and at the point of remand and sentence (Hood, 1992; Jones, 1985; NACRO, 1992); and within custodial institutions themselves (Genders and Player, 1989). Also, girls and young women in trouble did not benefit from the justice priorities of the new policy and practice consistent with their (white) male counterparts, remaining enmeshed within the vagaries of 'welfarism' and 'treatment' (Cain, 1989; Elliot, 1988; Harris and Webb, 1987; Hudson, 1988).

The prevalence of institutionalized injustice which underpinned the new juvenile justice policy and practice evidenced its partiality and structural tendentiousness. It could be argued that given time the principles of diversion, decriminalization and decarceration would have been applied comprehensively and equally to all children in trouble. This contention would amount to an expression of faith and optimism in the power and influence of the progressive juvenile justice practitioners operating within a liberal-democratic and consensual context. However, the consensual context was fragile. Indeed it was, as subsequent events have graphically illustrated, not a consensus at all but an expression of opportunism and political expediency. Despite the immense success of juvenile justice policy and practice during this period, and irrespective of the most unequivocal and convincing evidence, once its expedience was exhausted and the political priorities shifted, the fragility of the consensus was ruthlessly exposed.

The Post-1992 Clamp-down: A True Blue Approach to Children in Trouble

By early 1993 there was already a fermenting body of opinion that juvenile justice in particular, and penal liberalism in general, had gone too far. Since 1991 the media had taken a particular interest in teenage car crime and 'joyriding' and reports both sensationalized the nature of the offence and exaggerated its extent (Campbell, 1993). The 'joyrider' became the 'deathdriver' and the public were soon introduced to the 'ram raider'. Accounts of disturbances on the Blackbird Leys housing estate in Oxford, together with coverage of similar disquiet in Ely in Cardiff and areas of Birmingham became headline news. Televised scenes of children in balaclava hats apparently challenging and taunting the police with impish confidence on the Meadowell estate in North Tyneside were seen as live testimony of rampant mobocracy (Newburn, 1995). Next came the 'bail bandit' and the 'persistent young offender', children who were 'outside the law' and whose recalcitrance and disobedience was portrayed as being totally beyond the control of the courts and the police (Hagell and Newburn, 1994). This was not simply media hype, as it was afforded credibility and authority by public statements of the Association of Chief Police Officers (ACPO) and the reports of specific Chief Constables (Chief Constable of Northumbria, *Today*, 10 September 1992; ACPO, *Daily Mail*, 22 February 1993; Chief Constable of Dorset, *Daily Telegraph*, 17 June 1993). Throughout the 'consensus decade' the police and the courts had been hesitant, if not unwilling, partners and the Children's Society Advisory Committee notes:

> Police services in a number of areas released figures reflecting concerns about the increasing crime generally, and the problem of persistence. The police also submitted evidence to the House of Commons Home Affairs Select Committee, questioning the validity of claims that juvenile offending rates had fallen. Magistrates, too,

were reported to be resigning (13 in all) because of fears about the limitations on their powers, following the implementation of the Criminal Justice Act in October 1992 (1993:42).

There was little, if any, considered and dispassionate analysis during the frenetic months in late 1992 and early 1993 with no attempt to provide separate accounts for the different strands of youth deviance. A crude, reductionist assimilation of disparate behaviours was assembled and, in virtually no time, the consensus which had bound together over a decade of policy and practice developments began to crack. The conditions which would legitimize a complete repudiation of the principles of diversion, decriminalization and decarceration and an explicit rejection of what had been the government's position emerged at a furious pace. The tragic death of James Bulger in February 1993 and the subsequent arrest of two 10-year-old boys who were charged with his murder was shamelessly hijacked. The atypicality and extraordinary nature of this case was disregarded completely. It was portrayed as the ultimate expression of child lawlessness. A moral panic had been established and swift action was required if the 'new rabble' were to be prevented from marauding into 'decent areas' (Murray, 1994).

Such a moral panic was not unprecedented (Cohen, 1987; Pearson, 1983). However, no historical connections were made despite the Bishop of Worcester's observation that, 'It is not good enough for government or anyone else to play to the gallery and allow the media to manipulate us into a response that looks brave, tough and responsible, when in fact it is not any of those things . . .' (Children's Society Advisory Committee, 1993:7).

This is what happened as 'law and order has become a trophy with the political parties jockeying to show who is toughest on crime' (Kennedy, 1995:4). Within this context the lessons that had been learnt during the previous decade, and the need to recognize the distinctive characteristics of children and young people in trouble were submerged within cynical political posturing and authoritarian responses. In February 1993 the Prime Minister John Major proclaimed that, 'society needs to condemn a little more and understand a little less', and the then Home Secretary Kenneth Clarke referred to 'really persistent nasty little juveniles' (*Daily Mail*, 22 February 1993). The following month Kenneth Clarke announced to the House of Commons new proposals for 'that comparatively small group of very persistent juvenile offenders whose repeated offending makes them a menace to the community' (*Hansard*, 2 March 1993). Three months later, and after a Cabinet re-shuffle, Michael Howard made his first public pronouncement as Home Secretary, referring to a 'self centred arrogant group of young hoodlums . . . who are adult in everything except years' and who 'will no longer be able to use age as an excuse for immunity from effective punishment . . . they will find themselves behind bars' (*Daily Mail*, 3 June 1993). In October 1993, to rapturous applause at the Conservative Party Conference, Howard (1993) declared that he was speaking for the nation: 'We are all sick and tired of young hooligans who terrorise communities.' He promised a 'clamp down' and offered assurances that 'prison works'. The language and tone employed by the Prime Minister and his two Home Secretaries in describing children discharged contempt which was exceeded only by other senior colleagues, including David McClean and John Redwood. On television McClean was quoted as stating that 'our job is to drive the vermin off the streets' (*Panorama*, BBC1, 1 November 1993) and Redwood appealed nationally, 'Let us not call them ... disadvantaged youngsters or young offenders. Let us call them thieves, vandals and hooligans ... They are not prisoners of time and place. They should be prisoners at Her Majesty's pleasure if nothing else will stop them' (*Observer*, 24 July 1994).

During this period in 1993 the actual and real context of juvenile crime was lost within reactionary histrionics and authoritarian frenzy: the 'clamp down' was underway. 'Child criminals' suddenly became the 'enemies', the police had to mount a new 'war against crime', children and young people became 'beasts', 'evil', unprecedently 'wicked' and totally 'out of control' (Goldson, 1994:6). The conditions of moral panic were set. Genuine, albeit relatively uninformed, public concern was cynically exploited to legitimize the legislative backlash which served to dismantle and radically redirect the state's responses to children in trouble. Rutherford notes:

> Rapidly drafted legislation during 1993 shot great holes in the Criminal Justice Act 1991, which was shortly followed by the Criminal Justice and Public Order Act 1994. Where the 1991 Act had removed 14-year-olds from the prison system, the 1994 Act seeks to create a new generation of child prisons for 12–14 year olds. This is not a return to the 1970s but to the period preceeding the Children Act 1908 (1995:58).

Indeed, the 1993 Criminal Justice Act, which was hastily formulated within months of the implementation of the 1991 Criminal Justice Act (October 1992), served to re-establish the admissibility of previous convictions in relation to adjudications of offence seriousness which has particularly unfavourable implications for juvenile offenders. Moreover, the specific sections of the 1994 Criminal Justice and Public Order Act relating to children introduced a fierce tone of punishment and retribution: the introduction of new institutions – secure training centres – privately run for the purpose of incarcerating children as young as 12 years; the doubling of the maximum sentence of detention in young offender institutions; and the extension of the provisions of Section 53 of the 1993 Children and Young Persons Act relating to lengthy periods of detention for children convicted of 'grave crimes'.

Such draconian legislative change has been met with a barrage of informed critique from a wide range of academics, researchers, child welfare agencies and criminal justice organizations spanning the broadest political spectrum which, in turn, has been accompanied by expressions of deep concern from the churches. The Children's Society Advisory Committee (1993:38), commenting on the secure training centres, observes that, 'The Standing Committee on Youth Justice's statement of opposition was signed by 36 legal, child welfare, penal reform, health, education and youth work organizations.' Similarly, the Penal Affairs Consortium (1994:7), which comprises 23 organizations, concludes its case against the secure training centre as 'an expensive mistake . . . a sentence of detention in a new and separate system of secure institutions (run by commercial organizations with no experience of caring for vulnerable young people) is a step backwards in both penal policy and child care policy.' Further, opposition has focused on the 'Americanization' of the current policy direction in relation to juvenile justice. The odious and discredited 'three strikes and you're out' concept underpins the secure training centre, additionally, the government has established the first US style boot camp with a 'shock incarceration regime' for young people in trouble, despite evidence that the 'humiliating and degrading' punishment is an 'expensive failure' (*Guardian*, 14 March 1995; Penal Affairs Consortium, 1995).

Despite such authoritative and convincing opposition, however, the implementation of the legislation is underway. A second boot camp is planned (*Guardian*, 8 May 1995), the tendering process for the provision of five secure training centres in England and Wales has commenced (Howard League, 1995a:8), the Home Secretary is reported to have consulted with the Secretary of State for Defence to consider the possible placement of young offenders in 'glasshouse' military correction training centres (Penal Affairs Consortium, 1996), and statistics show a significant increase in the use of imprisonment and custodial remands. The Howard League notes:

> Despite the fact that levels of offending have remained relatively stable over the past five years, there has been a 25 per cent increase in the use of imprisonment over the past two years. Young people constitute a disproportionate percentage of this increase with increasing numbers of 15- and 16-year-olds being remanded into adult prisons . . . overcrowding has become a serious problem . . . NACRO has conducted three surveys which show juvenile custodial remands have increased from 440 in the six months before the Criminal Justice Act 1991, to 566 in the six months following the Act, to 658 during the six month period, October 1993 to March 1994. In all an overall increase of 50 per cent (1995b:12, 20).

Within little over a year the juvenile justice policy and practice which achieved so much throughout the previous decade, and promised much more, in terms of a sensible, effective, cost efficient and humane response to children in trouble, was dismantled. What has taken its place is an ill-considered and reactionary 'justice' programme which manifests profound institutional contempt for children and their welfare and which is imperious in its disregard for years of criminological research.

The Authoritarian Shift: A Critical Analysis

The radical change of legislative direction and juvenile justice policy lays down a fundamental challenge to liberal-democratic rationality. How could such a successful system be so speedily supplanted by a set of targeted responses which arise from and rely on an overtly politicized reactionary conviction and expressions of simple faith in punishment and retribution? The contention is that the authoritarian shift has been underpinned by insidious processes of demonization and detention, dematerialization and decontextualization, despotism and disqualification, each of which has served to mystify the precise nature of juvenile crime and legitimize the pathologization and brutalization of an identifiable group of children.

The Processes of Demonization and Detention

The malevolence and contempt that senior politicians employed in describing children in trouble has been unprecedented. Children have been pilloried in the most base and vulgar sense and their childhood has been systematically reconstructed so that those who offend are identified primarily as offenders rather than children (Crisp, 1994, 1995). Children in trouble have been defined as 'different', 'alien', 'other', 'evil' and 'wicked'; they are children 'possessed', little 'demons' from lawless planets – the planet 'inner city' and the planet 'outer housing estate'. Graef vividly captures the process of demonization:

> In order to feel good about oneself, in order to feel that you are a 'goodie', other people have to be 'baddies' . . . World War II gave the population of allied countries a very clear sense of who the 'baddies' were . . . That carried on through the Cold War . . . because again there was an 'evil empire' in Reagan's words. The Soviets were 'the baddies'. When we ran out of Soviets, we had the Libyans and the Iraqis. In the UK Margaret Thatcher coined that extraordinary phrase 'the enemy within', to describe the miners who, prior to that, had a privileged position as the 'salt of the earth', respected by virtually everybody. Within weeks her notion of the enemy within had transformed their public image, and distanced them. It had put them outside the pale that defined people like 'us' . . . The key to the entire mystic structure for the past 40 years . . . has been that if Western democracy, triumphed over the evil empire, then the fairy tale would have a happy ending . . . What has happened in the last few

years is that these fundamental myths and fairy tales have come to sticky non-endings. It has left us with the need for a new enemy. I suggest that children, and young offenders in particular, are now that new enemy . . . We are not talking about justice here. We are not talking about ordinary discourse or concern . . . The government now plans to spend 100 million pounds on locking up a small group of persistent young offenders, demonised by a language more reminiscent of seventeenth century witch hunts than late twentieth century criminology . . . we are not talking about children here we are talking about demons (1995:1–3).

Indeed, the demonization of children has provided a new 'enemy within'. The miners of the mid-1980s have been replaced by the minors of the mid-1990s. The individual personalities of children have been anonymized and de-humanized, their 'childhood' abandoned and an invented 'depravity' and 'wickedness', threatening 'decency' and 'discipline', has been profiled and emphasized. 'Lawless children' require 'childless law' and the process of demonization has provided legitimacy for the authoritarian shift in juvenile justice. This has negated the vulnerability of children in trouble and recon-structed them in such a way that detention seems the only solution.

The 'clamp down' has belied and disregarded all previous experience and knowledge that has been developed in relation to the vulnerability of many children in trouble, their histories of disadvantage and their needs for particu-lar forms of care, support and protection. Hagell and Newburn (1994) refer to the 'chaotic' lives of many juvenile offenders characterized by 'high levels of stress, bereavement and family break-up'. Bottoms (1995) found, 'abnormally high levels of family breakdown' and 'contact with the official care system'. A manager of a secure unit informed the Howard League Inquiry team that, 'up to 90 per cent of the offenders I have worked with have been sexually abused at home' (Howard League, 1995b:14). Kennedy, in the preface to the same report, observes that, 'Behind this report are many stories of pathetic young lives. As soon as faces and histories are given to the young people who are steadily filling our youth prisons, one is left with an overwhelming sense of hopelessness and wretchedness of their prospects' (1995b:4). The process of demonization has masked this reality as some of the most disadvantaged children in contemporary society are warehoused in stark custodial institutions.

According to recent statistics, the UK locks up more children in its prison system than any other country in western Europe with one exception (Kuper and Williamson, 1993:1). Further, there are profound qualitative concerns about the appalling treatment and conditions to which detained children and young people are exposed. Prison service staff have no background in child care or welfare and their priorities are focused exclusively on containment and institutional security. Overcrowding is endemic and much of the building stock is antiquated (Kuper and Williamson, 1993; NACRO, 1995; Howard League,

1995b; Tumim, 1990). One of the Howard League Inquiry Commissioners wrote immediately after a visit to Hull Prison and Remand Centre in September 1994:

> I find it hard to describe exactly how awful I found it. The building lacks natural light almost completely. Landings are narrow, separated by flights of stairs and suicide nets . . . The building is quiet but sounds echo. Furniture and fittings are of poor standard, and often piled into inappropriate rooms . . . To me the young people looked confused and aimless (1995b:25).

The conditions to which children are condemned are inhumane, brutalizing and abusive. Not only is the physical infrastructure strained and totally unsuited to guaranteeing basic standards of safety and welfare but the everyday operational realities are underpinned by a culture of bullying, intimidation and routine self-harm. Children, it seems, are not only being locked up *as* punishment but are being detained *for* punishment.

It is ironic that at the time when a growing body of research and professional activity is addressing the damage caused to children by bullying, developing strategies to counter bullying behaviour particularly in schools (Department for Education, 1994), incarcerated children are exposed to the starkest forms of bullying and abuse. The recently retired Chief Inspector of Prisons has drawn attention to the widespread nature and dangers of bullying and intimidation in custodial institutions (Tumim, 1992). His concerns have been echoed by the Prison Officers Association (House of Commons Home Affairs Committee, 1993). Moreover, the Howard League (1995b) reports, in the words of children and young people themselves, innumerable harrowing accounts of routine and systematic bullying in a wide range of custodial institutions. Such abject cruelty against children would not be tolerated in other settings and it is this vivid contradiction which exposes the dichotomy between state responses to deserving children and undeserving demons.

It is not surprising that many children and young people detained in prison custody experience significant difficulties, struggling to cope with their sense and experience of permanent fear and risk. The incidence of self-harm and suicide comprises the most striking reminder of the conditions to which children are exposed and directly connects with bullying and intimidation (Liebling, 1992; Liebling and Krarup, 1993). There were record levels of suicide and self-harm in youth custody during 1994 (Howard League, 1995b:14; *Independent*, 30 August 1994). In creating and maintaining these inadequate and dangerous institutions, the state abdicates its responsibility to children and, ultimately, to the public. The Howard League observes:

> an approach which concentrates on incarcerating the most delinquent and damaged adolescents, in large soulless institutions under

the supervision of staff with no specialist training in dealing with difficult teenage behaviour, is nonsensical and inhumane . . . the environment in which they are held can do little more than contain them like animals in a zoo . . . millions of pounds are being spent each year, producing increasingly damaged and recidivist young adults, whose ability to cope with normal life and engage in positive relationships has been dramatically reduced by the process of institutionalisation . . . The present direction of government policy is away from a unifying concept of childhood. Young people who have broken the law are dehumanised (1995b:67, 100).

The Processes of Dematerialization and Decontextualization

The period from 1979 to date has been marked by an intensification of socio-economic stratification and the emergence of deeper and wider forms of polarization and structural inequality (Hutton, 1995; Joseph Rowntree Foundation, 1995). Even government departments have provided unequivocal evidence that the gap between those with least and those with most has widened (Department of Social Security, 1993). Such economic patterns have inevitably impacted on children, with over 20 per cent now living in poverty (Oppenheim, 1993), 12,000 per day going hungry because there is insufficient money within their families to buy food, one and a half million living in overcrowded and unsuitable housing, and two and a quarter million school age children working illegally (NCH Action for Children, 1995:6). These children are bombarded with images of consumerist trappings and are growing up in a winner–loser society in which individual success is prized above all else. Yet they live in poverty and are not even provided with adequate food and shelter. Gross injustice and socio-economic disparities are not confined to individual families, they affect entire neighbourhoods, communities and sizeable geographical areas. It would be misguided and simplistic to proffer reductionist one-dimensional theories of anomie based on proposed causal relations between social disadvantage and juvenile crime. To ignore the material context, however, and reduce the analysis to the banal level of right versus wrong, decency versus depravity, and 'good' versus 'evil', in other words to get back to the basics of vulgar and decontextualized constructions of morality, manifests a crude and overtly ideological partiality. Yet this is exactly what has occurred as juvenile crime has been dematerialized within the 'clamp-down' conditions. Drakeford observes:

now this is very bad news indeed. Courts deal with the complicated human beings brought before them through a process of violent simplification. Taking one piece of a person's behaviour, removed from its wider context, and treating it as though emblematic of all that might be said of that individual forms part of the bedrock of the culture of severity . . . (1995:12).

The dominant discourse relating to children in trouble during the period of the authoritarian shift has been devoid of socio-economic analysis or any other consideration of the relationship between children and young people and public institutions. Many children experience a level of additional institutional exclusion which transcends and compounds existing structural exclusion. The emphasis placed on competitiveness, 'efficiency' and market imperatives has enveloped the entirety of public institutions. Concepts and policies such as local management of schools, parental choice, performance and attendance league tables have inevitably led to a hardening of attitudes which in turn has produced its casualties. Recent statistics show a sharp rise in exclusions within a relatively short period (Office for Standards in Education, 1993) with 19 children per day permanently excluded from their school (NCH Action for Children, 1995:7). While the relationship between school experience and juvenile offending is complex and unclear there appears to be some correlation between 'low achievement at school with higher delinquency rates' (Children's Society Advisory Committee, 1993:35). Graef notes:

British schools are excluding children well under 10 years old who are spending their time on the streets. What are we expecting those children to do with their energy, with their curiosity, with their time, or indeed with their lives? Excluding is the correct word, but we cannot exclude them from our community unless we spend 100 million pounds locking them up (1995:3).

But this is exactly what is happening. The National Youth Agency estimates that spending on the youth service nationally has been cut by 12.5 per cent over two years – from £240 million in 1991 to £210 million in 1993 (Children's Society Advisory Committee, 1993:35). It is ironic that the annual revenue costs for providing secure training centres are estimated at £30 million per year (Children's Rights Development Unit, 1994:207) a figure which exactly matches the swingeing cuts imposed on the youth service!

For older children making transitions into adulthood, the future is bleak in an increasingly unequal society in which they are at the sharp end of the collapse in paid employment and the abandonment and decimation of public housing with the consequent miseries of homelessness and destitution (Ashton *et al.*, 1990; Bates and Riseborough, 1993; British Youth Council, 1992; Williamson, 1993). It is established that entire sections of a generation of young people will experience long term unemployment and will be coerced into attending short-term and low-paid training schemes since the withdrawal in 1988 of their eligibility to claim state benefits and any entitlement to income support. The sense of abandonment experienced by 16- and 17-year-olds is percolating down as younger children witness the position of older sisters and brothers and realize what awaits them. Reductionist aetiology is flawed but the connection between the impoverished material context in which increasing numbers of children and young people are expected to survive and their delinquent behaviour cannot be ignored. Stewart and Stewart (1993) investigated the socio-economic circumstances of nearly 1,400 young offenders and provided a 'picture as bleak as anything that Dickens could have recounted'. Nearly three-quarters lived in poverty, one in five was homeless or threatened with homelessness, one-third reported going without food, a quarter were without necessary clothes (defined as one change of clothing and adequate protective clothing) and a quarter had inadequately heated homes or were without proper bedding. The report concludes that for many young people survival was the imperative behind their offending.

Given the evidence it is remarkable that the principal government debates comprising the dominant discourse have consistently dematerialized juvenile crime. Moreover, it is unacceptable that the government which has seemingly dispensed with an identifiable section of children and young people, a new surplus populace, is responding to their plight by warehousing them in custodial institutions. Drakeford writes:

> at a time when the social circumstances of people are so precarious so the calls from those most responsible for that predicament become most shrill and insistent. We live in an age of penal barbarism in which the most voracious and vengeful criminal justice system in Western Europe has as its most vociferous message that beggars must be swept off the streets because they are an offence to tourism and where the yob society is most piously attacked by those who have done the most to create the conditions in which it flourishes (1995:10).

The Processes of Despotism and Disqualification

The wealth of research findings that informed juvenile justice policy throughout the 1980s and into the 1990s demonstrated that most juvenile crime was non-serious and opportunistic, that most juvenile offenders grow out of delinquency and that custodial disposals are expensive, damaging and entirely counter-productive. As David Faulkner, the Head of the Home Office's Crime Department between 1982 and 1990, stated in a televised interview (*Panorama*, BBC1, 1 November 1993) this influenced the non-custodial emphasis in responses to children in trouble for a decade:

> The guiding principle of much of the policy in relation to juvenile offenders was one of the minimum use of custody and that policy was

considered until very recently to have been successful in the visible reduction of known juvenile offending during that period.

Although the most recent research findings are consistent with the 1980s' evidence, the government's policy remains diametrically opposed to that which was seen to be so effective. Most juvenile crime remains non-serious (House of Commons Home Affairs Committee, 1993; Howard League, 1995b:18). Although there is evidence that some children commit several offences, their *repeated* offending should not be confused with *serious* offending (Children's Society Advisory Committee, 1993:28–9). Most children, even those described as 'persistent young offenders' grow out of their anti-social behaviour (Hagell and Newburn, 1994), and custodial responses to children are not only inhumane but are more likely to confirm delinquent identities than deter juveniles from crime. On this point, informed opinion is consistent and embraces the widest range of positions including those of the churches and sections of the magistracy. The Bishop of Lincoln observes that, 'examination of past experience indicates clearly that jailing children has failed miserably' (Howard League 1995c:i). An editorial in *The Magistrate* concludes:

> Removing children from home, as a measure for reforming the individual, is a discredited policy. It does not reform; nor does it succeed in educational terms; it isolates children from their families; and when there are already adequate powers (though in some areas not the resources) with which to deal with the age group, it is horrendously expensive and wasteful of funds demonstrably better spent elsewhere in the juvenile justice system (February 1993:2).

Indeed, as Kennedy writes, 'Prison doesn't work. The claim that it does is no more than a crude slogan. The evidence shows it is not true but evidence no longer seems to be required in policy making' (1995:4).

Herein lies a dangerous facet of government policy regarding children in trouble: its resolute direction in the unequivocal face of contra evidence, its despotic drive, its disqualification of the legitimacy and its denial of research. The research evidence has not only been ignored but has also been withheld and dissent, however respectable, is being silenced. In mid-1994 the Dutch Ministry of Justice released figures indicating that juvenile crime in England and Wales was less prevalent than elsewhere in Europe (*Guardian*, 6 July 1994). It is extraordinary that the source of this information was an unpublished Home Office report, leaked to the British press by a Dutch government department. Later in the year the *Guardian* and *Independent* (28 August 1994) were the only national newspapers to cover a Government report which indicated that the number of known child offenders had fallen from its peak in 1985 (Government Central Statistical Office, 1994). In March 1995 Michael Forsyth, the Prisons Minister, attempted to suppress evidence compiled by civil servants concerning the expensive failure of American-style boot camps. Forsyth endeavoured to withhold the report from the House of Commons Library (*Independent on Sunday*, 19 March 1995). Moreover, the *Independent on Sunday* (8 January 1995) reported:

> The Home Office Research and Planning Unit, one of the most respected centres of academic crime studies in Europe, is being lined up for privatisation . . . A government-commissioned study on the possibility of contracting out the work of the 35 researchers – who, in the past, have attempted to ensure that government crime policy had a rational base – has concluded that the private sector could take over the unit's functions . . . Home Office union leaders alleged that the research unit was being punished for coming up with evidence that ministers did not want to hear . . . David Faulkner, a former senior Home Office advisor on crime, who is now at Oxford University, said: 'I'm afraid politicians are less interested in findings which do not conform with their dogmatic views' (8 January 1995).

Just as academic research has been expelled from the policy context, the processes of despotism and disqualification have undermined and marginalized professional discourse and crudely discredited developments in alternative practice in work with children in trouble. The creative, effective and sensible juvenile justice social work and probation practice which steadily developed between 1982 and 1992 has been discarded and considered professional perspectives have been ignored. Opposition to the secure training centres from *every* national child-care charity, professional associations, social services departments, the probation service, penal reform agencies, health, education and youth work organizations has been disregarded. Paradoxically, some of the staunchest resistance to these new jails for children came from prominent Conservative peers who moved a series of amendments in the House of Lords. In particular, Lords Carr, Elton and Allen moved that the Government would be creating 'schools for criminals' and that family ties would be seriously damaged (*Hansard*, 16 May 1994). Lord Carr, a former Home Secretary, had amendments supported in the Lords (*Hansard*, 5 July 1994) and the Government used its majority in the House of Commons to overrule the proposed changes.

Alongside the government's consistent rejection of professional opinion, social work has been caricatured, ridiculed and derided in the popular right-wing press. Stories of safaris and 'goodies for the baddies' have been grossly exaggerated as social workers have been maligned and pilloried as 'soft soaping do-gooders'. However, the prevalent antipathy to any notion of welfare in relation to 'offenders' is most evident in the government's targeted assault on the professional foundations of the Probation Service and its proposed arrangements for probation training and recruitment (Home Office, 1995). In turn it disregards the findings of its commissioned review (Dews and Watts,

1994). The government's review team engaged the broadest consultation, canvassing opinion concerning the efficacy of the system for educating and training probation officers. All 55 probation services, 34 universities and colleges, the Central Probation Council, the Association of Chief Officers of Probation and the Joint Universities Council–Social Work Education Committee were invited to express their views and 'argued strongly that the present arrangements met the service's needs' and should be maintained (Dews and Watts, 1994:2). Similarly, the Industrial Society 'thought the present arrangements quite effective' (1994:47). However, despite the findings of the detailed review, the Home Office announced:

A shake-up of the training and recruitment of probation officers . . . Lady Blatch said 'The probation service is moving into a new and increasingly demanding area and I want to see people who can respond to these challenges and who will be equipped to deal with the demands of the modern probation service' (1995).

The agenda was exposed by *Independent on Sunday* (8 January 1995) with reported Michael Howard's plans to 'fill the probation service with ex-army and police officers (as) . . . probation officers learn too much about racial discrimination . . . and the present recruitment system is leading to too many young women being hired'. The disregard for published research and attempts to withhold and silence material which questioned government policy, together with the negation of professional opinion and the determined assaults on probation education and training and the erosion of welfare perspectives, were not accidents or anomalous mistakes but integral elements of the processes of despotism and disqualification. The final element of these processes is the government's chauvinistic insularity and contemptuous indifference and disdain towards its obligations as provided by the United Nation's Convention on the Rights of the Child and related European instruments.

World-wide, 169 countries ratified the United Nation's Convention on the Rights of the Child which sets out principles and detailed standards for the treatment of children, for laws, policies and practices which impact on children, and for both formal and informal relationships with children. It has been accepted more quickly and more comprehensively than any other international convention, and 'UNICEF is seeking universal ratification by the turn of the millenium' (Children's Rights Development Unit (CRDU), 1994:xi). In September 1990 the World Summit on Children assembled in New York, constituting the largest gathering of world leaders in history. They included Margaret Thatcher and they pledged (1994:xi): 'The well-being of children requires political action at the highest level. We are determined to take that action. We ourselves make a solemn commitment to give high priority to the rights of children.' The UK government ratified the United Nation's Convention on the Rights of the Child in December 1991. The Convention is binding on the government under international law and it is obliged to comply with its provisions. The Government, however, from the outset, has been cautious as the Children's Rights Office (CRO, 1995a:18) notes:

> in the UK, international treaties are not automatically incorporated into domestic legislation. This means that it is not possible to use the domestic courts to challenge breaches of rights contained within the Convention. This can only happen if Parliament passes legislation which specifically incorporates its provisions. The UK government takes the view that no such legislation is necessary because the principles and standards of the Convention are already covered by existing legislation.

Two years after ratification there is a requirement on each government to send a report to the UN Committee in Geneva, the body elected to monitor and scrutinize the implementation of the Convention. The UK government's report was submitted to the UN Committee in February 1994 after the Department of Health had been given the responsibility for co-ordinating its production (Department of Health, 1994). The process of excluding professional opinion and expert perspectives again was in evidence, as the Children's Rights Office explains:

> In December 1993, the DH sent out a draft report to a limited number of organizations for comment. This was the first communication from the DH on the report. No prior discussion had taken place as to the key areas of concern in respect of children's rights or to proposals as to where legislative or policy change might be needed to achieve full implementation. The organisations were given eight working days over the Christmas period in which to respond to a document which was 100 pages long (CRO 1995a:19).

Contemporary juvenile justice policy in England and Wales runs contrary to the overall spirit of the UN Convention and to some of its principal articles, most notably Article 37 which states that 'the arrest, detention or imprisonment of the child . . . shall be used only as a measure of last resort and for the shortest appropriate time' (United Nations, 1989). This is consistent with three related international instruments to which the Government is formally committed: The United Nations Standard Minimum Rules for the Administration of Juvenile Justice: The Beijing Rules (United Nations, 1985); The United Nations Guidelines for the Prevention of Juvenile Delinquency: The Riyadh Guidelines (United Nations, 1990); and The United Nations Rules for the Protection of Juveniles Deprived of their Liberty 1990. Thus, unsurprisingly, in January 1995 the United Nations Committee reported violations of children's rights in the UK. The *Guardian* (28 January 1995) reported:

> Policy after policy 'has broken the terms of the UN Convention' . . . a report of the UN monitoring committee adds up to a devastating

indictment of ministers' failure to meet the human rights of Britain's children . . . the report is not all bad . . . however, the 'positive aspects' cover only four paragraphs, and the remaining 39 are either critical or are recommendations for action [which include] . . . abandoning the plans for secure training centres for 12–14 year olds . . . it also explicitly calls for 'serious consideration' to be given to raising the age of criminal responsibility.

The Committee's authoritative report comprises a clear, albeit measured, condemnation of the UK's treatment of children in trouble. Its findings should have triggered a Ministerial re-examination of the impact of government policies on some of the most structurally vulnerable members of society. The UK government, however, has not shifted its authoritarian position. Of the 32 signatories to the United Nations Convention on the Rights of the Child assessed by the monitoring committee only the UK government has refused to institute a parliamentary debate (Howard League, 1995b:97). Neither the summary record of the discussion nor the findings have been published or disseminated and the government, when asked about proposed action in response to the findings stated that nothing would be done (CRO, 1995a:25). Nowhere is the government's self-appointed omnipotence and unaccountability, in terms of its treatment of children in trouble, more apparent. John Bowis, the Under Secretary of State for Health, responded, 'Our track record is second to none. There is little that needs to be changed or improved in order to comply with the Convention. Other countries are beating a path to our door' (CRO, 1995a:25). The despotic tendency which underpins the policy direction in relation to juvenile justice was succinctly articulated in the *Daily Mail* (28 January 1995): 'How dare the UN lecture us. Failing our young? That's codswallop.' The legitimacy of the UN Committee in particular, and the Convention on the Rights of the Child in general, has been disqualified by the government in its unrelenting determination to clamp down on children.

Reclaiming Justice for Children: The Challenge Ahead

The effective and humane juvenile justice policy of the 1980s and 1990s which was underpinned by the principles of diversion, decriminalization and decarceration has been dismantled and replaced by a new get tough approach. The authoritarian clamp-down, which is directing contemporary state responses to children in trouble, has not gone unchallenged. Irrespective of the source of the challenge, however, it has been rejected at ministerial level. The government has positioned itself beyond the traditional boundaries of liberal-democratic accountability in its determination to punish children. It has severed the research–policy relation. It has attempted to conceal evidence which questions its priorities and it has posed veiled threats to non-compliant researchers. It has peripheralized professional discourse, ridiculed alternative approaches and introduced a crude disciplinary-correctives orientation to the Probation Service at the expense of its social work traditions. Remarkably, it has placed itself at odds with international opinion and abandoned its conventional obligations in accordance with European treaties. The government's despotic approach has disqualified dissent in a bullish pursuit of an authoritarian juvenile justice agenda. There is no rational criminological justification for the authoritarian shift. All of the available evidence from the broadest range of sources points to the counter-productive nature of the contemporary policy direction with its unwavering commitment to incarcerate greater numbers of children. By moving beyond the traditional boundaries of liberal-democratic accountability the 'clamp-down' is adrift and is careering towards the most ruthless assault on children and their childhoods for over a century. It is a brutal, symbolic expression of a hardline ideology within which the power to punish transcends any concept of child-care and child-protection. It is a painful reminder that reactionary political priorities eclipse rhetorical constructions of child-welfare and juvenile justice. Ultimately, it is an abdication of the government's responsibility to an identifiable group who are amongst the country's youngest and more defenseless citizens.

Kennedy (1995:4) observes that, 'the attitude we take to crime, and especially juvenile crime, is an important gauge of the kind of society we live in and the direction in which we are moving.' In this sense, contemporary state responses to children in trouble comprise both a chilling gauge and a foreboding sense of direction. The get tough policies which are grounded in common sense and claim for themselves populist appeal also resonate with a great simplicity which is unmistakably authoritarian. Such responses characterize a society within which all children and young people are structurally vulnerable, and those in trouble are particularly exposed to its disciplinary excesses.

As the new millenium approaches, the challenge that confronts those who share a concern in securing welfare and justice for children and young people is formidable. At the level of criminal justice it includes re-establishing, consolidating, and developing proven, sensible, effective, humane and cost-effective decarcerative policies and community-based practices. It necessitates a comprehensive reassessment of the juvenile justice system drawing on international experience, framed within European treaties, and giving particular consideration to increasing the age of criminal responsibility, abolishing the use of Prison Department custody for all children and young people, diverting resources from institutional settings to community-based programmes, and reserving Department of Health-managed secure accommodation for the relatively small number of children and young people whose behaviour places themselves and others at risk of significant harm. Juvenile/youth justice policies and practices must be subjected to permanent interrogation comprising both independent research and evaluation, internal monitoring and analysis. The findings from such scrutiny should be widely disseminated and applied in order to maintain and develop best practice and to inform strategies to eradicate institutional injustices from within the justice process.

On the macro-level, the reorganization of the juvenile justice system should be placed alongside a rigorous re-examination of the structural positioning of children and young people in relation to primary social institutions: their families, schools and communities. Social policy and institutional practices need to emphasize inclusion and recognition as opposed to exclusion and alienation. Co-ordinated corporate and inter-agency strategies at both central government and local government levels have to address the deepening poverty and material, cultural and social disadvantage that besets growing numbers of children and young people. Opportunities will need to be provided for children to contribute to the debates and their perspectives should inform policy and practice formulation. The state has to invest in children's futures providing enduring and meaningful opportunities. Such redirection will be the substance of a more heartening gauge. Politicians, together with social and economic commentators, may question the affordability of implementing such a programme. The question might be reframed: can any society which claims to value children, welfare and justice afford not to?

Chapter 7

'Mad', 'Bad' or Misunderstood?

Vicki Coppock

Children's behaviour, its definition, assessment and regulation, is rarely out of the news. It remains the focus of both professional and popular discourses, constantly labelled and regularly invoking calls for greater intervention. Within the ensuing debates the 'mad', 'bad' or 'sad' child is publicly defined and rarely consulted. Invariably, the public and professional debates turn on the conflated issues of 'acceptable' behaviour and 'normality'. The process of defining, identifying, explaining and responding to deviant or abnormal behaviour becomes the vital reference point against which normality is itself defined. What has emerged is a process, in both professional and popular discourse, based on binary opposition. Yet it is an arbitrary process which sets boundaries around normality without reflecting on historical, cultural, ideological, socio-economic and political contingencies. What follows is a critique of this process as it relates to children and young people whose behaviour is defined as 'disturbed' or 'disturbing'.

While clinical studies have attempted to give scientific rigour to judgments about disturbed or disturbing behaviour in children and young people, they rely heavily on adults – parents and professionals – to make initial judgments which determine particular behaviours as problematic. Thus, 'we have to see clinicians in their social role as authoritative interpreters of disturbance, adding a further layer to the common-sense definitions used by parents' (Grimshaw and Berridge, 1994:8). As Steinberg (in Malek, 1991:44) states, 'The process by which adolescents become psychiatric patients has as much to do with the feelings and behaviour of other people, and with social customs and routines, as with anything happening inside their heads'. This is not to deny that many children and young people experience mental distress. Nor is it suggested that parents and professionals are engaged in a conspiracy of ill-will. However, the medical model of mental health, which dominates the theory and practice of child and adolescent mental health, requires scrutiny in terms of its reliability and validity as an indicator of that distress. Such scrutiny is essential given the extent to which the medical model is utilized in professional interventions which impact significantly on the lives and opportunities of children and young people. Central to the dynamics of professional knowledge and practice is what Hood-Williams (1990) refers to as 'age patriarchy' – the way in which a range of elements including theoretical knowledge, institutional sites, legal codifications and professional practices structure the experiences of children and young people.

From an initial historical and theoretical contextualization of constructions of the mental health of children and young people, this chapter explores the problematics of the defining process, and its consequences, in the form of inconsistent institutional responses. The implications of differential interventions for the rights of children and young people are important issues here. Contemporary debates concerning the perceived deterioration in the mental health of children and young people are critically examined, along with official proposals for a coordinated child and adolescent mental health service. Finally, it is necessary to consider fundamental changes in adult–child power relations as the basis for creative and appropriate future policies and professional responses.

Historical and Theoretical Contexts

It is not possible to comprehend the significance of contemporary understandings of 'disturbed' and 'disturbing' behaviour in children and young people without reference to individual and, in particular, developmental psychology as the key framework of explanation. Theoretical knowledge and professional discourse emanating from psychology and psychiatry have stood as arbiters of normality and abnormality since the latter half of the nineteenth century. Individual psychology emerged in the context of late Victorian 'scientific' inquiry. Scholars of evolutionary theory, anthropology and philosophy, obsessed with numbers, measurement and quantification, searched for social laws to explain human behaviour. As part of this positivist tradition, child study – observing, weighing and measuring children, documenting their interests and activities – reflected the increasing importance of science. Not only did this tradition provide a set of procedures for conducting research, but also a set of practices associated with the modern state (Burman, 1994). Rose (1985) highlights the centrality of individual psychology in the role of classification and surveillance. Gradually, common-sense assumptions were translated into scientific truths, creating the context for, and giving legitimacy to, increasing practices of social regulation and reform. The emergence of individual psychology, at least in part, formed a response to wider social and political concerns of the late nineteenth century (Donzelot, 1980; Foucault, 1977; Rose, 1979, 1985, 1989, 1990). The consequences of early capitalist production, rapid industrialization and urbanization, produced unprecedented social upheaval, human squalor and misery. Fear of civil unrest was a real concern to the upper and middle classes, given the precedent set by the French Revolution. Fuelled by the 'scientific' rhetoric of Social Darwinism, attention focused on the physical and mental/moral 'quality' of the general population. Having discovered the principles of inheritance, there followed the possibility of the degeneration of the population through bloodlines and the 'overbreeding' of the poor, criminals, the physically and mentally disabled (Sapsford in Clarke, 1993). The fusion of the 'mental' and the 'moral' was crucial, 'to the extent that the object of political anxiety and scientific intervention became the "feeble-minded", who came to signify physical, moral, mental and political disintegration' (Burman, 1994:13). The stage was set for psychology to offer the 'tools' necessary for the identification, classification, control and regulation of those identified as threatening the social order. The establishment of compulsory schooling provided the psychologists with living laboratories in which they could observe large numbers of children (Rose, 1990). A mass of data was collected, standardized and analysed to construct norms for childhood growth and development. Mental testing provided an instrument through which normal or abnormal mental health and/or ability could be assessed and established. Yet, as Erica Burman observes, 'The normal child, the ideal type . . . is a fiction or myth. No individual or real child lies at its basis. It is an abstraction, a fantasy . . . a production of the testing apparatus that incorporates, that constructs the child, by virtue of its gaze' (1994:16).

Moreover, the practice of scientific research was dominated by the preoccupations and priorities of white, middle-class men, so that what became known about children and childhood carried assumptions implicit in patriarchy, colonialism and capitalism. Walkerdine comments that the coincidence of interest between the emerging profession of individual/developmental psychology and the wider political context cannot be reduced to some causal determination but 'each should be taken as mutually implicated, making and remaking each other possible, intertwining to produce a discursive and political nexus' (1984:173).

For Prout and James (1990) three themes underpinned the construction of the 'normal' child – rationality, naturalness and universality. Rationality is taken as the hallmark of adulthood, reinforced by a false ideology of childhood irrationality and incompetence. Just as femininity cannot be conceived outside its subjugation to masculinity, so childhood has been constructed as an inferior binary opposite to adulthood. Such assumptions have confirmed and legitimated the powerlessness of children by asserting their incapacity. 'Naturalness' and 'universality' provide the key ideological feature of inevitability, leaving little or no room for contradiction or conflict. The 'normal' child takes on an eternal, timeless quality, so embedded in the general consciousness that it becomes impenetrable. Consequently, the premises on which it is based – white, western, middle-class, male – have seldom been exposed, let alone challenged. Ultimately, such conceptions fail to acknowledge a variety of social relations and determining contexts within which children and young people are located.

A range of theoretical models of human behaviour has emerged from the late nineteenth century onwards. They coexist and compete with each other, tending to polarize around the nature v. nurture debate. The search for the 'x' factor, that which distinguishes 'normal' people from 'abnormal' people, has embraced such diverse issues as poor parenting (i.e. mothering), faulty social learning, biochemical imbalance and genetic structure. What they each have in common, however, is a focus on individual, familial and/or social pathology, and the overarching application of the 'medical model'. As Hargreaves (in Ford, Mongon and Whelan, 1982:35) explains, the medical model approach adopts 'the whole conceptual apparatus of symptom, syndrome, diagnosis, aetiology, pathology, therapy and cure'. While research has demonstrated a wide discrepancy between the criteria used for the identification of 'problem behaviour' and the assessment of individual cases, thus confirming 'fundamental disagreements between the professions over issues as basic as the definition of a disorder or the concept of treatment' (Hersov in Kurtz, Thornes and Wolkind, 1994:3), the medical model conveniently disguises these disparities. It is in the acceptance of a specific behaviour as a problem, an illness to be treated, that the power of professional hegemony is located. Once agreement has been reached, the only point of professional debate is *which* treatment should be given, *when* and *where* (Ford, Mongon and Whelan, 1982).

The medical model generates a polarized understanding of mental health rather than one which recognizes human behaviour as richly diverse and fluid, better represented as a continuum. It also fails to acknowledge that knowledge is not produced, nor do professionals practice, in a vacuum. 'Race' and gender characteristics, for example, clearly demonstrate the operation of subjective assessments in this field (Fernando, 1991; Russell, 1995). Discourses around femininity and masculinity have produced gendered constructions of 'acceptable' and 'unacceptable' behaviour for girls/women and boys/men. While 'for boys, aggression, assertion and delinquent behaviour are deemed natural, part of their progressive development ... [for girls] ... any deviance has been viewed as a "perversion" or the result of individual pathology which rejects passive, naturally feminine behaviour' (Coppock, Haydon and Richter, 1995:29–30). Similarly, an examination of the history of psychology and psychiatry illustrates the way in which ethnocentric and racist thought and practice has permeated these disciplines (Fernando, 1995). Negative stereotypes of black and ethnic minority children and families in Britain have been incorporated into the knowledge base and practices of professionals, constructing them as 'pathological' and 'deviant' (Dominelli, 1988; Hall *et al.*, 1978; Rooney, 1987; Torkington, 1983).

The role of the state in relation to child health, welfare and education has been well-established through a mushrooming network of institutions and academic/professional disciplines – medicine, psychology, psychiatry, health visiting, teaching, social work. Although each profession has developed within its own distinct institutional framework, professional practices have 'converged' at the site of discourse and 'knowledge' derived from within 'the psychology complex' (Rose, 1985). While it has been acknowledged that services for children and young people have been far from unified, evolving unevenly and without coordination, a professional hegemony can be identified within which the lives of *all* children and young people have been constructed through the dominant discourses of development and socialization. Foucault (1977) refers to these as 'regimes of truth', inscribed in the working practices of such professionals.

By the turn of the century in education there was a growing concern over 'difficult' children. Any children unable or unwilling to avail themselves of the 'cultural riches' of the established schooling system was assumed to be suffering from some form of 'mental defect' and thereby in need of segregation from 'normal' children. By 1907 the medical profession was firmly established within the apparatus of the Board of Education. The new body of school doctors (School Medical Service) became involved with 'defects' and 'disorders' of all kinds, bridging the medico-sociological divide. Nationally, the Chief Medical Officer (CMO), via his annual reports, played a significant role in early classifications of problem behaviour in pupils and the subsequent development of the child guidance movement of the 1920s and 1930s. In his 1927 report the term *maladjusted* was used for the first time, along with an account of his visit to a number of child guidance clinics in the USA. By 1929 the CMO was offering advice on the staffing of similar clinics in Britain, using the US multidisciplinary model combining psychiatry, psychology and psychiatric social work (Ford, Mongon and Whelan, 1982).

It was during the post-war period that the most significant advances were made in state responses to 'disturbed' children and adolescents, heavily influenced by the theoretical developments of Winnicott (1957) and Bowlby (1951). 'Maternal deprivation' was cited as a primary determinant of psychopathology in children and young people – a convenient message to all those women 'surplus to requirements' in the employment market. Women's futures lay in motherhood as their children's mental health depended on it. Singer concludes that, 'through the child, the mother was made responsible for violence and social chaos in the world outside the family, a world from which she was more or less excluded' (1992:99).

As child guidance clinics expanded throughout Britain, so did hospital-based child psychiatric clinics. The former were run by local authorities and had much closer links with communities and schools, while the latter were within the remit of the new National Health Service, attached mainly to paediatric services. Further, school psychological services emerged, reflecting the increasingly central role of educational psychologists in special education assessment. Further developments continued to be sporadic and were subject to considerable local variation. Additionally, there were significant differences in structure, function and therapeutic models.

The extensive reorganization of local government and the health service in 1974 was intended to streamline provision. By 1986, however, the NHS Health Advisory Service (HAS) reported patchy, uncoordinated services with children and young people falling through the net, an absence of planning and a tendency towards buck-passing between health, education, social services departments and voluntary organizations. The latter reflected increasing financial pressures on public sector services from the late 1970s and the swingeing cut-backs of the 1980s. The 'who pays' question began to dictate priorities, policy and planning. In 1986 the NHS Health Advisory Service Report optimistically recommended comprehensive, well-integrated services, joint inter-agency philosophies, planning and strategies. It offered a blueprint for creative development but this was not to be realized. Progressive tightening of public finance, education reform and local management of schools (1988 Education Reform Act), health service reform and the creation of the 'contract culture' (1990 NHS and Community Care Act), the burgeoning demands of child protection work (1989 Children Act) and community care implementation on local authority social services departments each militated against the development of any coherent and consistent national policy and coordinated practice regarding child and adolescent mental health.

The Problematics of the Defining Process

While theoretical developments and changes in practice imply a journey of innovation and progress in this field, critical research reveals this to be a misleading assumption. The historical vagaries concerning definitions of 'disturbed' and 'disturbing' behaviour in children and young people, when set alongside the structural inconsistencies in service development, clearly expose the scope for significant professional discretion and autonomy in decision-making processes. Although constructions of 'normality' and 'abnormality' have been firmly institutionalized in the state's response to children and young people, the catch-all nature of the formal diagnostic labels used allows for a wide interpretation of 'disturbance', from lying and disobedience to attempted self-harm (Jaffa and Deszery, 1989). For example, the Tenth Revision of the International Classification of Mental and Behavioural Disorders (ICD-10 WHO 1992 in NHS Health Advisory Service) states:

> Disorder is not an exact term, but it is used here to imply the existence of a clinically recognizable set of symptoms or behaviour associated in most cases with interference with personal functions. Social deviance or conflict alone, without personal dysfunction, should not be included in mental disorder (1995:17).

Yet the diagnostic classification of *conduct disorders* persists in child and adolescent mental health practice (see Kurtz, 1992; NHS Health Advisory Service, 1995). Clinical features cited include stealing, lying, disobedience, verbal or physical aggressiveness, truanting from school, staying out late, smoking, drinking and drug-taking. Moreover, it is widely acknowledged that conduct or behaviour problems are the most common presenting problem of childhood and adolescence, to the extent that it is feasible to argue that such 'problems' are statistically normal. For example, the Elton Report (Department of Education and Science, 1989) *Discipline in Schools* noted that 97 per cent of primary and secondary teachers reported 'disruptive' behaviour in their classrooms (i.e. talking out of turn; hindering other pupils; making silly noises; work avoidance; not being punctual; getting out of seat without permission). Similarly, the 1986 NHS Health Advisory Service Report (cited in Malek, 1991:8) notes that 'many of these behaviours might be regarded as an extension of normal adolescent behaviour but had been unacceptable...' Significantly, Rutter (1977), one of the most prolific writers and researchers into child and adolescent mental health, has stated that nonconformity can never be used as an indicator of psychiatric disorder and that psychiatric treatment has little to offer in cases involving 'disorders of conduct'. This brings into question the validity of diagnostic labels and the reasons behind the ongoing 'treatment' of substantial numbers of children and young people under these classifications. The circularity of definition is exemplified in one of the most recent studies on the prevalence of child and adolescent mental health problems and disorders (Wallace *et al.*, cited in DoH/DFE, 1995) where mental ill-health in children and young people is defined as 'a disturbance of function in one area of relationships, mood, behaviour or development of sufficient severity to require professional intervention.' Within the medical model, therefore, the presence of certain behaviours are simultaneously taken to signify the existence of, being also the consequence of, some abnormality.

The claim to specialist knowledge is central as it underpins the professionals' claim to be qualified to know better than clients, to be trusted by the public and to be given rewards and prestige, with significant powers of intervention (Williams, 1993). 'Expert' control distances parents and children through the use of technical jargon, a vocabulary which confuses and often predetermines outcomes through a subscription to categories or disease models. For parents the model has attractions in that they can feel relief at receiving an explanation for their child's behaviour which absolves them of the charge of 'bad parent'. For professionals the model allows them to be 'caring' while also repressing deviance, through the provision of help or treatment. In both cases the constraints of the model allows adult definitions of 'acceptable' and 'unacceptable' behaviour to prevail, leaving little room for any alternative understanding of the behaviour as an appropriate or reasonable response to stressful relationships between adult(s) and child/young person. For this is a relationship rooted in wider structural relations.

Research examining agency intervention in the lives of children and young people classified disturbed or disturbing (Malek, 1991) identifies the involvement of four main systems – education, social services, health and criminal justice. Substantial numbers of difficult children and young people have been located in residential care facilities of various kinds (Bebbington and Miles, 1989; Parker, 1988; Grimshaw and Sumner, 1991; Department of Health, 1992). Moreover, research indicates that each of these systems broadly deals with the *same* types of behaviours (Malek, 1991; NHS Health Advisory Service, 1986). As Malek states:

Many of the characteristics of young people which are perceived as making a significant contribution to their admission to psychiatric care are similar to those presented by young people who come to the attention of legal, educational, or social services authorities. This is particularly true of those who are admitted primarily for behavioural and/or emotional problems (1991:41).

Similarly, the 1986 NHS Health Advisory Service Report *Bridges Over Troubled Waters* notes that, more than any other client group, services for adolescents overlap many agencies, statutory and voluntary. Each system, however, assigns its own diagnostic label or definition derived from the historical vagaries and precedents of its particular professional knowledge base/ discourse. Consequently a child or young person could be given the label of *emotionally and behaviourally difficult* (education – special needs); *beyond parental control* (social services); *conduct disordered* (health – psychiatry); or *young offender* (criminal justice). This research not only demonstrates the arbitrariness of the processes through which 'disturbed' and 'disturbing' behaviour in children and young people is defined by parents and professionals, but also reveals how the diagnostic label and its application is contingent upon the first point of contact, identification and referral. Thus, the defining process is as much a cause of concern as the definitions employed.

The process is regularly set into motion following parental complaints concerning a child's or young person's intolerable behaviour. Typically, this includes disobedience, lying, staying out late, running away, truancy, theft, verbal and/or physical violence (see Grimshaw and Berridge, 1994; Jaffa and Deszery, 1989; Steinberg, 1981). Where help is sought invariably determines the route to provision. If pursued through the family doctor or health visitor, the 'problem' is diagnosed within a medical framework, most likely following the route to child and adolescent psychiatry. If pursued through school, it is given an educational focus and referred to an educational psychologist. Within social services, it is likely to be defined as a social/legal problem, depending on whether or not the child or young person has committed an offence. In Malek's (1991) research, professionals revealed that diagnoses are often made for administrative and bureaucratic reasons and do not always give a realistic indication of a child or young person's situation. Certainly, it does not follow that routes to provision are the result of rational assessment and planning as implied by the medical model. Moreover, within each system and at each stage of the defining process, assessments of behaviour operate within the determining contexts of race and gender, producing fundamentally different patterns and outcomes for girls and boys, and for black and white children and young people (see Cain, 1989; Campbell, 1981; Children's Legal Centre, 1994; Grimshaw and Berridge, 1994; Harris and Timms, 1993; Harris and Webb, 1987; Hudson, 1983).

Once 'the problem' acquires the status of requiring 'expert' intervention, things can be done to children and young people that otherwise would not be possible. The 1981 and 1993 Education Acts allow for formal assessment and statementing and for the removal of children and young people from home for residential special education. The 1989 Children Act, the 1991 and 1993 Criminal Justice Acts and the 1994 Criminal Justice and Public Order Act also allow for their removal from home to be looked after, remanded or serve sentence in the care of the local authority. Finally, they can be admitted to a residential psychiatric facility simply with parental consent, or under the provisions of the 1983 Mental Health Act. Not only is the process governing the 'system' through which children and young people are processed arbitrary, but also the implications of differential treatment between systems are far-reaching as each system offers them different legal rights. While general concerns have been expressed about safeguards guaranteeing the protection of rights, especially as a wide range of institutional and personal abuses have been identified in all settings, the work of the Children's Legal Centre (1991, 1993, 1995), Hodgkin (1993, 1994) and Malek (1991) has revealed how the mental health system offers children and young people the least protection from such abuses.

The Rights of Children and Young People in Residential Mental Health Settings

Interventions in the lives of children and young people because of their perceived 'disturbed' or 'disturbing' behaviour can escalate into a spiral of increasing restriction. Many children and young people find themselves in residential mental health settings either because of a lack of resources within one of the other local authority systems (Malek, 1991) or because one of the other systems considers them too disturbed for their intervention (Ivory, 1991). Once in this system, measures of control take on an overtly medical focus.

Critical analysis within psychology and psychiatry has acknowledged and shown the ease with which oppressive control can be redefined as 'therapy' (Edelman, 1977). This is particularly poignant for children and young people defined as 'disturbed' or 'disturbing', given the predominantly paternalistic framework which governs child welfare interventions. Prominent cases reflecting routine practices of institutional abuse and neglect have highlighted the thin line between methods used to control children and young people and the rhetoric of therapeutic intervention in their best interests (Children's Legal Centre, 1991, 1993; Fennell, 1992; Ivory, 1991; Ogden, 1991). For example: the 'pin-down' regime of solitary confinement used extensively in Staffordshire children's homes between 1983 and 1989; the physical abuse inflicted on children and young people at the Aycliffe Centre for Children by staff who had been trained in restraint techniques by officers from a local top security prison; the use and forcible administration of sedative drugs for control purposes at Hill End adolescent psychiatric unit, Langton House mental nursing home for children, and St Charles and Glenthorne Youth Treatment Centres. Such cases reveal how, in addition to the routine practices of behaviour modification, seclusion or solitary confinement, psychiatry utilizes an even more powerful method, that of drug therapy. From this evidence it has become clear that the treatments directed towards 'difficult' or 'disturbing' behaviour within the mental health system often have grave consequences for the civil liberties of children and young people (Hodgkin, 1993, 1994).

Although children and young people in mental health care can be afforded protection under the 1983 Mental Health Act if they are 'formal' patients, more than 90 per cent are admitted 'informally' by their parents or the local authority looking after them (DoH, 1986). Often the term *informal* is incorrectly substituted by the term *voluntary*, constituting a serious misnomer. As Stewart and Tutt argue:

> there is a sense in which all children in mental hospitals are hidden in custody because they are not allowed to discharge themselves without their parents' consent and nearly always it was their parents, or occasionally care authority, who originally requested admission (in Malek, 1991:5).

In these settings there is no legal framework within which the rights of children and young people can be safeguarded, particularly in relation to the restriction of liberty, consent to treatment or complaints procedures. There is no access to Mental Health Review Tribunals, nor do they come within the scope of the Mental Health Act Commission. The Commission has expressed considerable concern about the lack of safeguards and has requested that its remit be extended to cover informal patients. Consequently, in 1990 the Department of Health issued a New Code of Practice in relation to the 1983 Mental Health Act. This was revised in 1993 to bring it in line with the 1989 Children Act. The purpose of the Code was to supplement the Act, offering practical guidelines and guiding principles around admission, consent to treatment and complaints procedures. However, there is no statutory duty attached to the Code. It applies to all patients, including those under 18. In relation to this age group the Code states that practice should be guided by the following principles:

- Young people should be kept as fully informed as possible about their care and treatment; their views and wishes must always be taken into account.
- Unless statute specifically overrides, young people should be regarded as having the right to make their own decisions (and in particular, treatment decisions) when they have sufficient 'understanding and intelligence'.
- Any intervention in the life of a young person, considered necessary by reason of their mental disorder, should be the least restrictive possible and result in the least possible segregation from family, friends, community and school (Children's Legal Centre, 1993:7).

The Children's Legal Centre (1991:24; 1993:3–6) has accumulated substantial evidence of practices which continue to give cause for concern:

- lack of knowledge and implementation of legal rights concerning consent to medical treatment, and a general lack of rights to self-determination;
- ongoing segregation outside mainstream institutions and schools, away from family, community and friends;
- discriminatory practices leading to unjustifiable intervention and detention on the grounds of class, race, ethnicity, gender, sexuality, disability, etc.;
- unnecessary restriction of liberty, use of restraint, locked rooms, seclusion, time-out, etc.;
- inadequate assessment and, thereby, lack of care;
- indiscriminate use of drugs to control rather than treat;
- inappropriate and degrading behaviour modification techniques – deprivation of sleep, food, clothing, family contact;
- ongoing placement of children and young people in adult psychiatric facilities;
- lack of rights to confidentiality and privacy;
- use of peer pressure/bullying to maintain discipline.

These practices demonstrate that professional practice does not reflect the spirit of the Code. Several commentators have asserted that it is the reliance on common law and discretionary guidance and the reluctance of professionals to *formally* detain children and young people under the 1983 Mental Health Act which leaves them exposed and vulnerable to human rights abuses (Bates, 1994; Fennell, 1992; Masson, 1991). It is a reluctance derived in the 1957 Percy Commission, which stated that children and young people should be admitted 'by the exercise of normal parental authority' (in Bates, 1994:133).

Since the 1969 Family Law Reform Act, however, 16- and 17-year-olds have had a statutory right to consent to medical treatment, and since the landmark ruling in *Gillick v. West Norfolk and Wisbech Area Health Authority [(1986) A C 112]*, those under 16 have had a statutory right to consent to treatment (without parental knowledge or consent) provided they have 'sufficient understanding and intelligence'. This ruling was thought to have marked a new era in relation to children's rights as it dismissed the idea that parents had absolute authority over their children until they reach 18. The Gillick Principle was evident in the 1989 Children Act, bolstered by the UN Convention on the Rights of the Child in the same year. A series of high profile cases, however, have cast doubt on the scope of the Gillick decision in relation to the right of a child or young person to refuse consent to treatment (Bates, 1994; Fennell, 1992; Freeman, 1993; Lawson, 1991; Masson, 1991). It had been assumed that a 'Gillick competent' child was entitled to give and to refuse consent to treatment. Yet the Court of Appeal decided that any person with parental responsibility, or the High Court with its inherent jurisdiction, in certain situations, is able to override a child or young person's right to refuse treatment.

The cases of *Re R, Re W and Re H* (cited in Bates, 1994; Children's Legal Centre, 1995; Fennell, 1992; Freeman, 1993; Lawson, 1991; Masson, 1991) each involved consideration of the compulsory treatment of 'disturbed' children and young people. In each case the right to refuse medical treatment was overridden. Moreover, their refusal to consent to treatment was taken as indicative of their 'Gillick incompetence'. Fennell suggests that this is problematic:

> What is not acceptable is the automatic assumption that refusal is irrational and can be overridden whether or not the patient is competent. This is the very assumption which underlies Lord Donaldson's guidance – that children under 16 are never competent, even if they are *Gillick* competent, to refuse treatment as long as someone else with a concurrent power of consent agrees to it (1992:327–8).

Adults are presumed to be competent unless there is evidence to the contrary. Thus, it is the severity of the test for 'Gillick competence' which 'provides the basis for decisions in individual cases which ignore the child's wishes' (Masson, 1991:529). From this, Masson deduces that it is virtually impossible to envisage a situation where a child or young person with a negative mental health label could ever refuse treatment. She challenges the paternalism inherent in the Court of Appeal decisions which allows adult views to dominate and suggests that this stems from 'the belief that paternalism is better than self-determination where decisions relating to children are concerned' (Masson, 1991:529).

The Current 'Crisis'

It is clear that the situation has become a legal minefield in which the debate is conducted exclusively by adults, leaving children and young people without a voice or the right to consultation. What small advances that had been made towards their involvement in decisions about their lives, respecting their views and enabling them to take greater personal responsibility, have been negated or exposed as rhetoric. This is of particular concern given statistical evidence demonstrating an alarming increase in the numbers of children and young people being admitted to residential psychiatric care. According to Rickford, Department of Health statistics show a 65 per cent increase in admissions between 1985 and 1990 for those aged 10 to 14 years, and a 42 per cent increase for those under 10 (*Independent on Sunday*, 4 April 1993). Thus, significantly more children and young people are experiencing the overtly medical, psychiatric system with all this implies for their civil liberties. Such a dramatic statistical trend warrants closer examination and an understanding of the context of change.

These statistics, coupled with intense media coverage of a number of high profile cases, such as the killing of James Bulger, have provoked extensive debate focusing on a perceived 'crisis' in the psychological health of children and young people. It is suggested that society is witnessing unprecedented levels of 'disturbed' and 'disturbing' behaviour in children and young people. Moreover, this alleged deterioration has been repeatedly connected to notions of increased violence and lawlessness. This is derived not only in the media and from the outbursts of politicians, but also in the statements of professionals who claim to work in the interests of children and young people. For example, Peter Wilson, Director of Young Minds, stated that, 'Most of us in the field agree that the degree of distress in young people is much more extreme now. They are exhibiting more extreme behaviour and are given to finding more violent solutions to their problems' (in Sone, 1994:16).

Similarly, Sue Bailey, consultant adolescent forensic psychiatrist, claimed to be dealing with 'slightly more psychotic children than two years ago' (Sone, 1994:16).

While such behaviour could be interpreted as indicative of greater resistance from children and young people, challenging adult social control, in reality the intertwining of the 'mental' and the 'moral', so evident in the Victorian understanding of deviance, has gained a new lease of life. Politicians across the political spectrum, social commentators and professional 'experts' have been busy with television, radio and newspaper specials devoted to the subject of whether children and young people are 'madder' and/or 'badder' than in previous generations. Explanations offered are varied but cover familiar ground as illustrated by the following quotes:

> I believe that human nature spurts out freaks. I believe these two are freaks and they just found each other (Detective Sergeant Phil Roberts, interviewing officer, Bulger investigation, *Public Eye*, 24 November 1993).

> Evil can creep up on children (John Patten MP, *Newsnight*, 24 November 1993).

> By the age of ten a child should have developed a conscience. By the age of ten some children's experience of life has left them without a conscience at all (Mark Easton, reporter, *Newsnight*, 24 November 1993).

> Unmet emotional needs lead to inadequate parenting and damaged children (Doreen Goodman, 'What About the Children?', *Guardian*, 22 February 1993).

> Jonathan, born in 1982, must have spent his first years in an atmosphere of tremendous maternal tension (Gitta Sereny, *Independent on Sunday*, 6 February 1994).

Since all children are highly impressionable, how can we possibly avoid some savage social penalty in later life? (Consultant psychiatrist, Parkhurst Prison, *Guardian*, 22 February 1993).

I've seen a growth in violent behaviour by boys who were brought up with no male figure. They feel close, dangerously close to their mothers and are frightened of it (Valerie Sinason, child psychotherapist, *The Sunday Times*, 21 February 1993).

Biological determinism, religious/moral degeneracy, attachment failure, maternal deprivation, environmental determinism, paternal deprivation, ill-discipline, bad teachers, broken homes, single mothers, video nasties, the list is almost endless. Those who support the assertion that there is a demonstrable increase in the mental ill-health of children and young people tend towards two distinctive explanations: those who blame the victim and those who consider children and young people as blameless victims of a deteriorating society. What they share, however, is the assumption of pathology. By contrast, Malek (1991) has challenged this notion of a crisis in the behaviour and mental health of children and young people. Her research reveals that many find themselves in psychiatric care due to a lack of resources within their local authority social services or education departments. As resources have diminished within these systems, so increasing numbers of children and young people spill over into the historically better resourced health system, giving the impression of an increase in madness.

This observation is supported by many practitioners. Dr Greg Richardson, consultant child and adolescent psychiatrist, commented, 'I have a lot more pressure to admit young people for problems previously dealt with by social services' (*Independent on Sunday*, 4 April 1993). The Association of Metropolitan Authorities expressed similar concerns (see Sone, 1994). Another consultant stated that between 60 and 70 per cent of the children in the psychiatric unit for which he had responsibility were there for conduct disorders rather than any specific psychiatric illness. He concluded, 'If they have not got an illness that is treatable, they do not belong in hospital' (*Independent on Sunday*, 4 April 1993). Nevertheless, the professional and political interest in the subject of child and adolescent mental health intensified in the wake of the perceived crisis. A series of official documents were published reviewing child and adolescent mental health services throughout all the relevant agencies (DoH/DFE, 1995; Kurtz *et al.*, 1994; NHS Health Advisory Service, 1995). A substantial overhaul of current provision was proposed involving 'the adoption of a coordinated, tiered, strategic approach to the commissioning and delivery of child and adolescent mental health services' (NHS Health Advisory Service, 1995:2). This recommendation was a response to the key findings of the review: 'that child and adolescent mental health services are essentially unplanned and historically determined; that their distribution is patchy; that the work being done is variable in quality and composition; that the work they do seems unrelated in strength or diversity to systematically considered local need' (1995:3).

The key proposal was to establish a four-tiered service. Tier 1 includes professionals who represent the first point of contact between a child or young person and their family and child-care or health agencies such as GPs, generic social workers, teachers, police, school medical officers, school nurses and health visitors. It is intended that these professionals provide access to the more specialized services by explicit routes negotiated and instituted locally. Tier 2 consists of interventions by individual specialist child and adolescent mental health professionals such as community psychiatric nurses, psychiatrists, clinical psychologists, educational psychologists, psychiatric social workers, psychotherapists and occupational therapists. It is envisaged that these staff will also provide support, consultation, education and advice to staff at Tier 1. They will also act as gatekeepers for access to services at Tiers 3 and 4. Tier 3 consists of interventions by teams of the specialist child and adolescent mental health professionals identified above. It is expected that these staff will bring coordinated interventions to more complex problems which cannot be managed at Tier 2. They would act as gatekeepers to the highly specialized services of Tier 4. Tier 4 provides for specialized interventions and care, for example, out-patient mental health services; in-patient mental health services; special units; secure forensic mental health services. The proposals also include joint assessment of population needs, individual needs, agency needs, research and development needs, and staff training needs; joint agreement of strategy; joint service planning; joint care planning, care management and care programming; joint purchasing; and joint evaluation and monitoring.

If such a model is to be effective it will require significant resourcing. Further, it will demand that the various systems dealing with the 'disturbed' and 'disturbing' behaviour of children and young people, with their different agendas, ideologies and languages, put aside their professional rivalries and interests. To date such an ambitious task has proved unattainable (NHS Health Advisory Service, 1986). What is fundamentally different, however, is the strong business management emphasis in all contemporary documentation. The language of the market is all-pervasive: purchaser/provider; clinical audit; rational planning; joint commissioning.

Further, Keegan Eamon's (1994) critique of state responses to child and adolescent mental health in the USA signals a worrying trend which could be replicated in the UK. Calls for coordinated services and comprehensive networks have been virtually ignored by the federal government and public services have been subjected to massive cutbacks and decline. Instead, the market-place has been allowed to flourish and dictate 'appropriate treatment' for children and young people. The rapid growth of 'for-profit' child and adolescent mental health establishments is the main reason for the dramatic increases in the institutionalization of children and young people in the USA. Typically, those classified as rebellious, disruptive or non-compliant make up the expanding populations in such institutions (Weithorn in Keegan

Eamon, 1994). Inevitably this has impacted significantly on the lives of black children and young people, already over-represented in such classifications. In some states, the staff in these establishments determine what is 'medically necessary' for a child or young person, exposing an inherent conflict of interest when profits are dependent on admissions. While the UK experience has not yet reached this state of affairs, the signs are not reassuring. For example, private tendering for the provision of secure training units for 12- to 14-year-old children provides a clear indicator of the political direction, driven by free-market, economic libertarian imperatives.

Challenging Professional Discourses and Classifications

Throughout the twentieth century, concerns have been continually expressed about the behaviour of children and young people, eliciting persistent responses from the state via a range of professional interventions. Yet, there is a sense in which the contemporary 'crisis' reflects an intensification of a much wider moral panic around childhood. This implies that it is adults' fear of the loss of their control, the loss of their power over children and young people, which is at the heart of the much-proclaimed 'crisis'. Psychological and psychiatric 'expertise' has inspired panic in adults about childhood, predicting catastrophe from the slightest parental 'mistake'. It has cultivated a belief in the ability to know, understand, predict the course that 'normal childhood' should take. It is this claim that has been found wanting, understandably leaving lay adults bewildered. Through critical research and analysis the hegemony of professional discourses around mental health which underpin and legitimate adult power over children and young people has been exposed as at best spurious and at worst overtly oppressive. The definition and demarcation of mental 'health' and mental 'ill-health', of 'normal' and 'abnormal' childhood(s) are riddled with social and political meanings.

The established political or professional rhetoric cannot disguise the fact that the UK government's commitment to the holistic well-being of all children and young people is inadequate, fragmented and under-resourced (Calouste Gulbenkian Foundation, 1993; Children's Rights Development Unit, 1994; Hearn, 1995; UN Committee on the Rights of the Child, 1995). In this context it is hard to envisage a fresh, enlightened approach to the mental health needs of children and young people. Rather, the proposed changes to improve partnership and collaboration between purchasers and providers in child and adolescent mental health services (NHS Health Advisory Service, 1995) could merely facilitate a further attempt to consolidate professional hegemony, contributing to the long history of policy, legislation and practice in this field which has served to strengthen adult control.

There remains a desperate need to construct new ways of responding to children and young people in distress. The Children's Legal Centre points to the lack of 'ordinary' people and places to whom they can turn when they are distressed. It is suggested that there needs to be 'a shared and common responsibility, not merely within the obvious statutory, voluntary and private agencies, but throughout society to enable children and young people to receive the advice and help they need' (1991:25). In this sense a positive approach to the mental health needs of children and young people can be achieved only in the context of a wider change in adult–child power relationships. This demands that children are respected as people first, that they are listened to and that they have the right to make informed decisions about their lives, free from adult judgments concerning their competence to do so. Practitioners need to acknowledge that while their practice is grounded in the traditions of the medical model of mental health they will fundamentally fail children and young people. They must retreat from institutionalized 'age patriarchy', which involves the abuse of knowledge and power. Moving on means dealing with the messy contradictions inherent in adult–child relationships. It means asking questions, recognizing inadequacies and challenging oppressive structures. Only then can adultism be deconstructed and the human rights of children and young people respected.

Chapter 8

Whose 'Childhood'? What 'Crisis'?

Phil Scraton

Childhood is mapped by rituals imposed from above. From the moment of birth, through family and community induction, religious and cultural initiation and on to the seemingly unquestioned gradation of formal schooling, the baby–toddler–child is celebrated and processed through the ritualizing of his or her progress. The progression of the person-in-the-making or adult-in-waiting is predominantly temporal. Children are 'big/small for their age' or 'ahead of/behind their class/grade'. They are 'backward', 'forward', 'slow', 'quick', 'gifted' and classified. Until recently, and still present in popular discourse, such classifications included 'handicapped', retarded or educationally subnormal. Common-sense and popular assumptions dovetail with institutional practices and policies in conferring appropriateness as 'childhood' behaviour and its progression is subjected to routine assessment. The scrutiny and classification to which they are subjected is not restricted to physical growth and academic attainment. Dress, manners, speech, hair, jewellery, beliefs, style, music . . . the list is endless. Each is measured against standards imposed by those adults significant in children's lives and they are regularly reminded of the consequences of a 'bad attitude' or mixing with the 'wrong people'. Their gullibility and corruptibility is taken-for-granted and emphasized. Within this context children's experiences are reconstructed by adults who easily portray power as responsibility, control as care and regulation as protection. Typically, adults direct and children obey, with age and status (parent, guardian, professional) ensuring legitimacy.

The ritualization of childhood, steeped in the symbolism of celebration, maps the 'progression' of the child through his or her stages of development. At the level of appearances the moments of celebration, from birthdays to prize-givings to religious ceremonies, are child-centred. Yet they function also as adult-defined practices of conformity. Beginning with initiation into familial, community, religious, cultural and institutional practices they become profound processes through which children are socialized and conditioned. Deviation from the charted path inevitably leads to condemnation, punishment and even expulsion (from school, from church, from home). Within this context of discipline, regulation and correctionalism, passive or active resistance by children and young people is always defined as negative, as a challenge to legitimate authority. Perhaps the most disturbing feature of the control imposed on children, both in formal institutions and in informal interaction, is the overarching and shared assumption that left to their own devices children lack collective responsibility, run wild and destroy each other. Writing only days after the death of James Bulger, for example, Melanie Phillips and Martin Kettle commented '. . . it begins to seem that William Golding's fictional universe of juvenile savagery in *Lord of the Files* lies all around us in our housing estates and shopping malls' (*Guardian*, 16 February 1993). As noted in Chapter 2, Golding's fiction is taken as a pseudo-scientific cautionary tale that children abandoned or bereft of the discipline and guidance of adults will sink to unknown depths of cruelty and individualism normally avoided by the civilizing process of adult society. What an incredible irony this represents given the apparently insatiable appetite that much of the adult, patriarchal world has for violence, brutality, war and destruction.

Deliverance from 'Evil'

As a process of normalization, the ritualization of childhood is about power relations. The socialization of the child and the definitions of appropriate development are not open to negotiation, except between 'knowledgeable' adults. This text provides a mass of contemporary evidence, derived in a wide range of children's experiences, which consistently demonstrates the silence of their voices, the absence of their feelings, the neglect of their needs and the denial of their ideas from political debates, institutional decision-making and policy initiatives which shape their lives. The regulation and control of children's behaviour, that which amounts to the imposition from above of disciplinary power, is effective precisely because of its invisibility, its taken-for-granted legitimacy. As Foucault (1977) maintains, the most effective exercise of power is that which operates through 'subtle coercion'. It is not simply that adults conspire to exclude or marginalize children and young people from the processes of consultation, decision-making or institutional administration but that there is no conceptualization or recognition that such processes might be appropriate. What this amounts to, however, is a coincidence of adult interests across all institutions in both the private and public spheres.

Children and young people have always posed problems for the adults in their lives yet there remains the much-promoted and oft-quoted myth, usually based on childhood reminiscences of the defining adults, that there was once a 'golden age' of compliance and discipline in which authority prevailed and every child knew its place. The idea that childhood deviance, youth lawlessness and anti-authority attitudes have escalated and are indicative of a broader moral decline within a previously stable and conforming social order is enduring. Each generation progressing through parenthood and into middle-age cannot remember a time when children were so ill-disciplined and so dismissive of their elders. Pearson (1993/94:190) quotes a range of sources which indicate that harking back to an earlier period of 'civility and order when the traditions of family and community were still intact' has become a regular British pastime. He quotes a Christian youth worker, James Butterworth, writing in 1932, as bemoaning the 'passing of parental authority, defiance of pre-war conventions, the absence of restraint, the wildness of extremes, the confusion of unrelated liberties, the wholescale drift away from churches . . .' (1993/94:190). In 1930 F. R. Leavis talked of the 'vast and terrifying disintegration of social life' with catastrophic change destroying the family; 'the generations find it hard to adjust themselves to each other . . . parents . . . helpless to deal with their children' (1993/94:190). 'We have arrived', wrote T. S. Eliot, 'at a stage of civilization at which the family is irresponsible . . . the moral restraints so weak . . . the institution of the family is no longer respected' (1993/94:190). Roy and Theodora Calvert identified a national 'crisis in morals'. Pearson closes his discussion of the inter-war years with a quote from A. E. Morgan in 1939:

> Relaxation of parental control, decay of religious influence, and the transplantation of masses of young persons to new housing estates where there is little scope for recreation and plenty of mischief . . . a growing contempt for the procedure of juvenile courts . . . The problem . . . is intensified by the extension of freedom which . . . has been given to youth in the last generation (1993/94:191).

Pearson is insistent, and the evidence is convincing, that the 'same rhetoric' which is 'utterly misleading in its emphasis on the novelty and unprecedented dimensions of juvenile crime', has been employed for over a century. He concludes:

> The fact that we seem to be able to persuade ourselves in the 1990s that we are passing through an unprecedented crisis of public morals, while expressing our fears in a language which is indistinguishable from that of generations which are long dead, is an extraordinary historical paradox which reflects an equally extraordinary historical amnesia about even the more recent past (1993/94:191).

What Pearson's work shows is that the grand delusion of an 'unprecedented crisis of public morals' has remained a persistent feature within popular discourse throughout the twentieth century. The issue is not simply that the past is forgotten, but that it is idealized. Undoubtedly, there has been an increase in community tensions, anti-social behaviour and the fear, if not the reality, of crime. The disruption of community identities and their social cohesiveness has contributed to a range of predatory and threatening behaviours as loosely-defined and poorly-serviced communities turn in on themselves. But there is a tendency to interpret the back-to-back nineteenth century neighbourhoods, the impoverished tenements and the twentieth century under-resourced redevelopments as honourable environments virtually free of disruption, disorder or mischievous children.

Just as Pearson's work illustrates the extent and depth of adult indignation as each ageing generation wrings its hands at the declining moral fibre of its children, so the process is renewed, often in more measured published or broadcast commentaries. In July 1994, for example, *The Sunday Times* published an article by Gerald Warner on the 'ills' of contemporary childhood which encompassed the full range of reactionary opinion towards all things progressive. He centred his analysis on childhood in Scotland and warned 'Civilisation menaced by adolescents from hell' (*The Sunday Times*, 3 July 1994). His starting point was the James Bulger case which established his key themes:

> What I did on my holidays the 1994 version. Put concrete block on railway line, am; abducted toddler from supermarket and beat him to death, pm. Who said that today's youngsters do not know how to make their own entertainment?

Quite apart from representing one of the most untypical crimes of the decade as typical, almost casual, these opening lines trivialized a tragic case and, on its back, condemned a generation of children. Warner warmed to his task: 'releasing the school population into general circulation [school holidays] is a life-endangering exercise.' Why? Because it is a population of 'sullen, introverted, ignorant and loutish young people' who threaten the 'future of our country' and 'civilisation itself'. A 'nation of vipers' has been bred whose 'prevailing ethos is anti-social' (*The Sunday Times*, 3 July 1994).

Warner's world is one of absolutes, a world in which 'political correctness' portrays children as the 'victims' of unemployment and poverty. Schools are 'appalling', denied the essential tool of discipline: corporal punishment. Teachers 'live under a regime of terror, fearing physical assault or false accusations of "abuse".' This, he argues, is evidence that the 'balance of power' in schools has been inverted. While teachers run scared, parents 'spawn' the 'monsters'. The political context of Warner's 'breeding-ground of anarchy' is 'two decades of political correctness' dominated and sustained by the 'Leftist thought police' who banned the works of authors such as Enid Blyton. But,

> Blyton children had two parents and fought crime; politically correct children should have one parent (or live with two homosexuals) and commit crime . . . 'The youth of a nation are the trustees of posterity,' claimed Disraeli. He was right; in this generation that is a terrifying thought (*The Sunday Times*, 3 July 1994).

Warner's article could be dismissed as being no more than a reactionary rant against progressive trends, the kind of contribution so much the stock-in-trade of Conservative Party Conference fringe meetings, occasionally spilling onto the main conference agenda. It cannot be so lightly passed over. For it represents the sharp end of a continuum of child rejection. It is a sharp end most accurately described as child-hate, in the same vein as race-hate, misogyny or homophobia. This form of argument takes an event which is atypical, in this case the killing of James Bulger, and represents it as typifying a generation lost to the basics of morality, discipline and responsibility. The hatred, apparently reserved for cases marked by exceptional and unusual cruelty and brutality, is extended to include a range of behaviours construed as offensive or anti-social. Thus the atypical transforms into the stereotypical.

What this rhetoric appeals to, and it has been successful in maintaining its constituency, is the notion of inherent evil. There is no shortage of reference points for this construction of the evil spirit lying dormant, waiting to be triggered, within the apparently innocent body. Christianity, for example, despite its diverse religions, holds steadfastly to the conceptualization of original sin and the intrinsically imperfect or flawed soul of the individual. It represents an ever-present feature of belief systems which implore that their 'faithful' be 'delivered from evil' and led 'not into temptation'. Further, the biological determinism of the early medical models of deviant behaviour, although challenged by rationalism, promoted the construct of inherent, if not inherited, evil. Rationalism, which argued that individuals knowingly and voluntarily took decisions to commit crime, become deviant or behave offensively, did little to challenge the proposition that evil originated within the individual. The conceptualization of 'evil' within the aberrant child has a long tradition with religious, academic and child-care institutions. It resides permanently beneath the surface which presents a veneer of tolerance and understanding in direct contrast to the forces released once children and young people step out of line.

The killing of James Bulger unleashed a level of adult vindictiveness unprecedented in recent times. Children suspected of the murder and taken into custody for questioning, despite their innocence, were unable to return with their families to their homes. Following their arrest, the two boys charged with the murder of James Bulger made court appearances marked by scenes of mass, adult hysteria. Hostile crowds attempted to break through police cordons to attack the vehicles in which it was assumed they were being transported. Once convicted, and following the trial judge's statement that their act was of 'unparalleled evil' (*Daily Express*, 25 November 1993), the press lost no time in presenting full-page photographs of the 'Freaks of Nature' (*Daily Mirror*, 25 November 1993). Another headline, 'How Do You Feel Now, You Little Bastards' (*Daily Star*, 25 November 1993) encapsulated and reflected on an adult nation's demand for revenge. As Chapter 2 shows, there was hatred evident in much of the public's response and the demand for the boys' execution. It was endorsed with enthusiasm by media coverage, a sense of moral outrage closely aligned to the demand for retribution. This process not only influenced the trial, the sentence and an intervention by the Home Secretary setting a minimum period for the boys' imprisonment (declared unlawful in

July 1996), but it promoted a severe backlash directed against progressive and successful youth justice – and other institutional – policies. The case became a metaphor for children's 'lost innocence' and the triumph of 'evil' over 'good'. Within five months Home Office Minister, David McLean, had the line 'our job is to drive the vermin off the streets' removed from a speech by his advisors.

The political reaction which followed the death of James Bulger, although rarely as vitriolic as Warner's later article or McLean's censored statement, reflected a broad consensus and some specific similarities. Within days of the murder the Prime Minister, John Major, called for a 'crusade against crime' and a 'change from being forgiving of crime to being considerate to the victim' (*Mail on Sunday*, 21 February 1993). While there was no evidence in the public domain of people being forgiving, particularly of the much-proclaimed misbehaviour and ill-discipline of children and young people, the Prime Minister was eager to regain the initiative in the law and order debate. Over the previous 12 months there had been continual media coverage of the supposed post-1960s liberalism and permissiveness which allegedly had dominated the youth justice and youth morality debates. The former had focused on alternatives to custody programmes, particularly those involving groupwork and rehabilitation at outdoor centres. Without any reference to the relative costs (diversionary programmes were significantly cheaper than custodial regimes), benefits or objectives of such programmes, they had been roundly dismissed as holidays or rewards for offenders. At the same time, as Chapter 6 shows, the Association of Chief Police Officers and other police organizations announced a crisis in youth crime, specifically centred on 'persistent young offenders' and joyriders. The message, endorsed by John Major, was that in order to redeem the harm done to victims of crime, there was required a return to harsher, punitive regimes geared to the disciplining of children and young people.

Kenneth Clarke, then Home Secretary, was unequivocal in his attack on 'persistent, nasty, little juvenile offenders' and their apologists. For him, they were indicative of 'a loss of values and a loss of a sense of purpose . . . partly due to a weakening of some of our institutions . . .'. He railed against social workers as 'not succeeding with children' concluding that 'it is no good mouthing political rhetoric, as some of them do, about why children in their care are so delinquent' (*The World this Weekend*, BBC Radio 4, 21 February 1993). This suggested 'loss of values', together with what was alluded to consistently as weak or permissive professional intervention, addressed the issue as one of moral philosophy rather than one of structural and material conditions. As the chapters on schooling and sexuality demonstrate, the political and media rhetoric suggested the moral degeneration of childhood, aided and abetted by irresponsible parents and liberal professionals. It was an issue taken beyond the confines of crime and offending behaviour to represent a multi-dimensional crisis in children's social identity and moral responsibility. Rather than the Labour Party opposition addressing concerns about the experiences, opportunities and frustrations of children and young people as a disenfran-

chised group facing the erosion of welfare provision, under-resourced schooling and diminishing work opportunities, its leaders appeared to mouth the
same rhetoric as Government ministers. In his submission to Labour's Commission on Social Justice the then Shadow Health Minister, David Blunkett,
echoed his Conservative counterparts:

> Those committed to a new twenty-first century welfare state have to
> cease what has been seen as paternalistic and well-meaning indul-
> gence of the sub-culture of thuggery, noise, nuisance, and anti-social
> behaviour often linked to drug abuse. Understanding the causes of
> decline is not the same thing as tolerating the consequences.

For Tony Blair, then Shadow Home Secretary and aspirant Prime Minister, recent events were 'like hammer blows against the sleeping conscience of
the country'. Learning and teaching the 'value of what is right and what is
wrong' offered the only safeguard against 'moral chaos' (*Guardian*, 20 February 1993). Labour policies, Blair argued, would challenge the 'moral vacuum'
and be 'tough on crime and tough on the causes of crime'. Noting its 'grave
disquiet at the growth of vicious and unprovoked attacks on the most vulnerable in society . . .' an all-party group of MPs tabled a House of Commons
motion locating the crisis in 'a decline in standards of personal responsibility
and respect for others' (*Hansard*, 19 February 1993).

Conveniently ignoring the statistical evidence which showed that Britain
locked away more young people, earlier in their lives and for longer periods of
time, than any other European Union member state, the demands for punishment, retribution and deterrence became overwhelming. Sir Ivan Lawrence
QC, Chairman of the Home Affairs Select Committee on Juvenile Crime,
captured the reactionary spirit of the moment:

> There is a hard-core of persistent young offenders, and too many of
> them are simply laughing at authority and thumbing their noses to
> the court. The biggest punishment is simply to take away their free-
> dom. But they should also learn discipline and a respect for authority
> there (*Guardian*, 22 February 1993).

In October 1993 Michael Howard, the new Home Secretary, delivered his
uncompromising message to the Conservative Party's Annual Conference –
unveiling his 27 steps to 'crack crime'. In an atmosphere which drew sustained
and enthusiastic applause for a delegate's demand for execution, castration
and beating, headlined in *Today*, (7 October 1993) as 'Hang 'Em High, Hang
'Em Often', Howard reiterated almost word-for-word the earlier censored
statement of his under-minister, David McLean: 'we are sick and tired of these
young hooligans . . . we must take the thugs off the streets' (*The Sun*, 7 October 1993). His commitment, previously announced by Kenneth Clarke, was to
integrate into youth justice provision secure accommodation for 12–14-year-

old children. Added to this would be USA-style boot camps based on the principles and practices of military correction. Within months, James Bulger's death had become a catalyst for the consolidation of an authoritarian shift in youth justice. It was a shift which, in legal reform and policy initiatives, was replicated throughout all institutional responses to children and young people. It carried media approval and popular (adult) consent, reflecting the well-established Thatcher agenda of the 1980s.

The Social Construction and Political Management of the 'Crisis'

As previously discussed, the portrayal of 'dangerous children' or 'lawless youth' has remained a prominent feature of British social life over the last two centuries. Constructions of childhood rebels and delinquent gangs have remained high in the public consciousness, fuelled by associated moral panics and media amplification. Broader social trends or specific events at any moment, or in any given location, can only be fully interpreted through recognizing the social construction of reality in which popularly-held assumptions and media portrayals converge. As Chapter 2 illustrates so clearly, the media plays both a formative and a reflective role in this process of social construction. It mobilizes and reproduces images that have a resonance within its audience, reflecting and mirroring the prejudices, beliefs and anxieties that hold sway. Chomsky argues that in the 'manufacture of news', there is conformity to ideological pressures which reflect internalized values derived in structural power relations. He states:

> The system protects itself with indignation against a challenge to the right of deceit in the service of power, and the very idea of subjecting the ideological system to rational enquiry elicits incomprehension or outrage, though it is often masked in other terms (1989:9).

While Chomsky's analysis is concerned with the creation of those 'illusions' necessary to maintain the US state's credibility with regard to foreign policy and military interventions, the significant point is that the media not only reflects back to its audience that which is expected – patriotism, for example – but also that it endorses and underwrites the interests of the powerful within any given social order. It generates a subtle mix, appealing to constituencies of prejudice, manipulating – even inventing – 'the truth' and servicing, not always without mild criticism, established-order priorities. The communications' revolution has provided the media with unprecedented capacities to reach vast audiences in an instant. As photographs, reports, comment and televisual data flash around the world, courtesy of media conglomerates' satellites, new technologies secure the images in seconds and broadsheets are published in hours. With political futures won and lost on television presentations, with wars broadcast live into sitting-rooms and com-

puter-enhanced images of slow-motion, action-replays routinely used to identify the 'deviants', the power of the media to manufacture news has entered a
new, global era dictated by its attendant global market-place.

There exists a considerable body of primary research illustrating the
capacity, and apparent willingness, of the media to manipulate coverage to
satisfy political–ideological agendas or to win readership or ratings battles.
Within this broader context the media, particularly the press, has been culpable in the purposeful fabrication of stories relating to quite different events
or incidents. Examples such as coverage of the 1984–85 coal dispute (Wade,
1985), prison protests in Scotland (Scraton, Sim and Skidmore, 1991) or in
1991 at Strangeways, Manchester (Jameson and Allison, 1995) and the
Hillsborough Disaster (Coleman *et al.*, 1990; Scraton *et al.*, 1995) parallel the
coverage of St Saviours School, Toxteth, discussed in Chapter 2. The images of
'militant' trade-unionists, 'psychopathic' prisoners, football 'hooligans' and
'lawless' children were created without supporting evidence and sustained
over time, guaranteeing their acceptance without question. They appealed to
an already established constituency within the public domain where the 'language of law and order . . . sustained by moralisms' (Hall, 1979:19) has suc-
ceeded in delivering the syntax of 'good' against 'evil', the standards of
'civilized' against 'uncivilized' and the choice of 'anarchy' against 'order'.

It was the appeal to values and morality which cemented the Thatcherite
agenda bringing popular consent to the worst excesses of economic libertarianism and social authoritarianism. The media has played a significant part in
this process. As Herman and Chomsky state:

> the 'societal purpose' of the media is to inculcate and defend the
> economic, social, and political agenda of privileged groups that domi-
> nate the domestic society and the state. The media serve this purpose
> in many ways: through selection of topics, distribution of concerns,
> framing of issues, filtering of information, emphasis and tone, and by
> keeping debate within the bounds of acceptable premises (1988:298).

The 'privilege' enjoyed by adults when set against the experiences of children
and young people is their function as active participants, namely citizens,
within society. The media's participation in the social construction of reality is
framed inevitably around the marginalization and exclusion of children, reflecting a broad adult consensus around 'childhood', its social identity and
political management. The stories about children's behaviour which have
dominated the press throughout the 1990s represent a conscious blend of
imagery and ideology. Journalists and editors have taken the sensationalist,
dramatic images of troublesome children and lawless youth, regardless of their
accuracy, and touched the raw nerve of established ideologies. So strong are
the ideologies which prevail over crime, disorder and deviance, saturated with
dominant notions of 'evil', 'viciousness' and 'savagery' that the constituency
thirsts for the grotesque and the horrific. On the one hand is the moral

indignation of condemnation, harsh punishment and retribution, on the other is the amoral infatuation with the violent and brutal details of tragic cases.

Crime, disorder and deviance are part of a broader context of social construction in which images reflect shared and persistent ideologies. Popular assumptions about racial superiority and 'lesser breeds', deeply embedded in the English national psyche, and given credence by a century of eugenics, are regularly reinforced in media coverage of 'alien cultures' and immigration policy. Similar assumptions about 'problem estates' and 'sink schools', reflecting established class ideologies, are reinforced by media stereotypes of an underclass which inhabits 'no-go' areas. There are many examples which connect commonly-held assumptions based on internalized prejudices and bigotry to news coverage and political commentary within the media. Whatever the publishing and broadcasting guidelines require, the media is not in the business of education but in the business of news production, literally selling news. It is a cut-throat and competitive world in which the supply must be responsive to the demand. And truth, accuracy or enlightenment are often the first casualties.

The social construction of reality, manifested in and maintained by popular discourse, however, creates expectations and requires responses. If it constitutes a shared 'way of seeing', the political management of 'social problems' forms the basis for 'ways of responding'. The popular discourses outlined above have gained credibility from mainstream academic discourses and their 'domain assumptions'. 'Wayward children', 'dysfunctional families' and 'degenerate communities', whatever the tensions between competing theories, have been closely associated with an implicit, and often explicit, acceptance of pathological models. While early physiological theories of the 'deviant' or the 'delinquent' were overtaken by more refined theoretical constructs, focusing on genetic predisposition, and by the more socially contextualizing arguments of 'under socialization', the focus remained the same: individual pathology. Although quite different and distinct premises underpinned such models, ranging from biological/social determinisms to rationality and voluntarism, the emphasis remained consistent: the abnormal individual.

Similarly, the early sociological studies of the inner-city by late nineteenth century reformers, emphasized the corrupting influence of moral degeneration. Through the application of medical frameworks and analogies the social environment, or laboratory, was pathologized. In this construction people might not be born with criminality in their genes but they could be infected. As Mort (1987) so clearly shows, the medico-legal discourses of the late nineteenth century pulled together a range of quite unconnected social issues: poverty, sin, vice, crime and political sedition. From these early discourses emerged a growing academic analysis of environment and culture. Just as the body could be infected, creating a 'sick' person, so communities could be infected, creating a 'sick' society. Whatever the broader, structural relations of class, unemployment, poverty and appalling housing, the issue was reduced to morality. The political rhetoric and academic accounts fused together in their common assault on the 'idlers' and the 'unemployables' whose parlous state was represented as being of their own choosing. It was a fusion of like prejudices which remained almost untouched, and certainly intact, to be mobilized with a vengeance as the New Right of the 1970s invoked the 'Old Right' of the 1870s: the 'return to Victorian Values'.

The significance of medico-legal discourses which centre on some combination of individual and social pathology models – the bad, mad, sad individual or the bad, sick, infected and infectious community – is not only that they dignify and legitimate the bigotry of popular discourses but also that they actively promote policies of correction. For, if individuals or communities can be identified as being inherently pathological, they can be classified, targeted and disciplined accordingly. As Foucault (1977) demonstrates, in the pursuit of the 'disciplined subject' the regulatory functions of the 'professionals' become institutionalized. In this process Foucault's 'regimes of truth' are not dissimilar to Berger's 'ways of seeing' as prioritized 'social problems' become politically managed through state agencies. Knowledge might be diverse and differentiated but if it carries the weight of state agencies and their regulatory intervention it is knowledge interwoven with authoritative power. While power takes many diverse and relative forms, manifestly pluralized through complex social relations, in its political–economic forms it is persuasive. For those pushed to the political and/or economic margins, the relative surplus population and/or political activists, it is their personal or social worlds which become the focus of attention. Their actions are targeted, policed and regulated and their knowledge is contested, ignored and disqualified.

This is not to suggest that seriously disruptive, antisocial and criminal behaviours do not exist, are to be denied or can be reduced simply to political–economic determinants. Although, as Bea Campbell (1993) notes, it is no coincidence that young working-class men terrorize communities within a broader socio-economic context which presents the rhetoric of stake-holding while purposefully and institutionally denying their participation. It is also no coincidence that they are men behaving badly within patriarchies which make virtues of male aggression, bonding, camaraderie, homophobia and misogyny (Stoltenberg, 1991). While deeply offensive and threatening behaviours require appropriate policing, there is a lack of political will to examine and reform the structural, determining contexts which sustain the threats, the violence and the fear. It is not just a case of historical amnesia, as Pearson (1993/94) notes, but a remarkable reluctance to learn from history.

Consequently, authoritarianism, so much the hall-mark of Thatcherism, is not simply a populist dogma carefully orchestrated to win the hearts and minds of 'middle England'. It is the ever-present flip-side of the liberal, benign state. The social authoritarianism of the New Right has been unwavering in its commitment to the politics of correctionalism through punishment. In responding to individuals who transgress the law, the driving force has been a combination of punishment, retribution and deterrence. The popular appeal is that offenders 'get what's coming to them' and are compelled to conform through experiencing thoroughly unpleasant regimes of harsh punishment. At the community level the process of pathologizing identifiable families and groups has meant the growth of surveillance, targeting and regulation. What the pathology models suggest is a policy orientation towards normalization through correctionalism. This suits policies whose popular appeal is derived in demands for retribution and 'just desserts'. The political management of 'dangerous children' and 'lawless youth', then, reflects the social construction of 'dangerousness' and 'lawlessness' more broadly rooted in popular discourse.

Taking the Moral High Ground

Charles Murray, writing on the emergence of a British underclass during the 1980s, identifies three primary 'phenomena' which together form its structural foundation. These are illegitimacy, violent crime and drop-out from the labour force. 'Illegitimacy', however, constitutes the 'best predictor of an underclass in the making' (Murray, 1990:4). Murray's thesis is that children become 'responsible parents and neighbours and workers' because they copy the role models in their communities. Given that the 'responsible' community is one of 'appropriately' formed nuclear families with functioning parental roles, Murray's identification of dysfunction is as predictable as it is simplistic and crudely reductionist. It begins with an easily recognized stereotype, the 'lone mother', and quickly shifts to the pathologization of entire communities.

> A child [by which he means boy-child] with a mother and no father, living in a neighbourhood of mothers and no fathers, judges by what he sees . . . in communities without fathers, the kids [by which he means boy-kids] tend to run wild. The fewer the fathers, the greater the tendency . . . no set bedtime . . . left in the house at night while mummy goes out . . . an 18-month-old toddler allowed to play in the street . . . children who are inordinately physical and aggressive in their relationship with other children (Murray, 1990:11–12).

For Murray young men 'are essentially barbarians' and it is marriage, 'the act of taking responsibility for a wife and children' that is 'an indispensable civilising force' within society (1990:23).

Murray's thesis not only appealed to the New Right, it gained indirect support from self-styled realists on the liberal left, particularly ethical socialists. Prominent among the regular contributors to this debate is *Guardian/Observer* columnist, Melanie Phillips. Central to her argument is the pre-eminence of 'adult gratification' over the 'best interests' of children. Discussing the 'catastrophic failure of the parental relationship' Phillips argues:

> . . . the assumption that long-distance fatherhood is just another dish to be chosen from the menu of alternative family structures, the

peripatetic plight of children torn between two households, are ... familiar features now of everyday life. And their consequences are becoming all too familiar: the rising levels of childhood and adult distress in Britain, Europe and America, from depression and eating disorders, through educational underachievement, truancy and the flight from what is sometimes laughingly called home, into lives of homelessness, crime, drug abuse, failed relationships, suicide and despair (*Observer*, 13 June 1993).

Phillips shares with Murray the belief that settled marriage constitutes the 'civilising force' essential to societal stability and the primary socialization of children. For Phillips the 'crisis of the family' is a 'crisis in authority' and the 'attempt to rebuild a decent society will founder unless the two-parent family takes its place again as the template for a society based on co-operative, responsible and altruistic relationships' (*Observer*, 13 June 1993). Concluding that a father is 'a vital necessity for a child's emotional health', Phillips drives home her argument:

Two parent families ... are the model of a healthy society ... the cohesiveness of our society is at risk, too many of our children are in trouble and *all* parents urgently need help and support. We need to move from self-indulgence to social responsibility (*Observer*, 13 June 1993).

Phillips persistently returns to this social tension between 'self-indulgence' and 'social responsibility'. Writing on 'no-fault divorce', for example, she refers to criticism of 'pro-family campaigners' as embodying the 'increasing shrillness of the libertarian hedonistic tendency' (*Observer*, 29 October 1995). In discussing the case of Sarah Cook, a 13-year-old girl who married an 18-year-old Turkish national, she condemned it as a 'fitting take for the nihilistic nineties' (*Observer*, 28 January 1996). She railed against the 'astonishing' attitude of Sarah Cook's 'ordinary parents':

Their behaviour demonstrated a complete breakdown of any moral code whatsoever ... an utter failure to understand what parenting is ... It showed they had no concept of any values beyond immediate gratification ... (*Observer*, 28 January 1996).

'Self-indulgence', 'hedonism', 'nihilism' and 'immediate gratification' form the judgmental currency employed by Phillips in specifying a 'decline in family values'. As illustrated above, the repeated attacks on 'lone parents' or 'dismembered families' by the ethical socialists, together with those made by the New Right on 'illegitimacy', are instrumental in laying blame on specific individuals and communities. The tone of the writing assumes that those who endure misfortune, poverty and under-resourced environments make conscious choices to exacerbate their suffering. It is the perception of voluntarism so evident in this work that makes it so detached from reality. There is also what Ros Coward refers to as 'horrendous middle-class bigotry' as 'the problem then becomes the sub-human culture of the poor threatening to overwhelm fundamental human decency' (*Guardian*, 2 December 1994). As Suzanne Moore puts it:

> Flaunting one's idyllic marriage and achieving children does little to help those who have tried and failed, not because we are immoral, irresponsible people but because we are full of human failings and may have made wrong choices or felt that there was no choice to make . . . Pronouncements about the social good of the marital institution do little apart from propagating the idea that, when it comes to families, some are more equal than others . . . Children are suffering through material, not maternal or paternal, deprivation. This, for me is the real moral issue (*Guardian*, 9 March 1995).

Phillips' journalism, however, cannot be dismissed lightly as the writings of an individual, torch-carrying media commentator. It is well-respected and reflects a growing and influential constituency. She identifies closely with the writings of 'ethical socialists' such as Norman Dennis, George Erdos and A. H. Halsey and her work is consistent with the public statements of 'left realist' politicians such as Labour leader Tony Blair, and his shadow cabinet minister for education, David Blunkett. Dennis and Erdos (1992) take the debate away from the confines of Murray's inner-city underclass to propose a more universal, far-reaching social breakdown connecting 'illegitimacy' and family 'breakdown' to a reduction in the work ethic and spiralling crime. Halsey (Foreword: Dennis and Erdos, 1992:xi) argues that the traditional family provided a 'coherent strategy for the ordering of social relations in such a way as to equip children for their own eventual adult responsibilities'. Accepting that family life has been eroded he identifies (1992:xiii) an 'overlooked consequence' of 'family breakdown':

> the emergence of a new type of young male, namely one who is both weakly socialised and weakly socially controlled so far as the responsibilities of spousehood and fatherhood are concerned . . . he no longer feels the pressure his father and grandfather and previous generations of males felt to be a responsible adult in a functioning community (1992:xiii).

For Dennis and Erdos the lack of 'responsible fathers' is the persistent theme as 'young males . . . no longer take it for granted that they will become responsible fathers' (1992:27). Dennis, 'by the summer of 1993, under the pressure of the cumulative evidence from common experience and statistical evidence' had established 'beyond doubt the superiority, for the children and for the rest of society, of the family with two publicly and successfully committed natural parents' (1993:69). In attempting to sustain this position he quotes an article published in *The Atlantic Monthly*, a 'leading journal of the liberal-left' in which Barbara Dafoe Whitehead wrote:

> The social science evidence is in: though it might benefit the adults involved, the dissolution of intact two-parent families is harmful to large numbers of children. Moreover . . . family diversity in the form of increasing numbers of single-parent and step-parent families does not strengthen the social fabric but, rather, dramatically weakens and undermines society (1993:70).

Again, the emphasis is that adults, steeped in selfishness, nihilism and self-indulgence put their interests before the established 'needs of children' and the identified 'good of society'. For the ethical socialists it is a state of affairs encouraged by, and indicative of, a deepening social and moral shift supported by a post-1960s 'received wisdom'. Dennis and Erdos (1992:25) argue that such 'received wisdom' suggests that 'institutions which normatively held these areas [sexuality, procreation, child-care, child-rearing and adult mutual-aid] together in a tight inter-locking package [lifelong heterosexual socially-certified marriage] were "not deteriorating, only changing" '. As with Melanie Phillips, Dennis and Erdos propose that such a position constitutes a serious and sustained ideological attack on the family which collectively represents an 'anti-family consensus'. Underpinning this attack, and providing academic credibility to this subversive consensus are the 'betrayals' of the 'intellectuals': 'ad hoc combinations of destabilizing Marxism whose long march through the institutions began and ended in the family, altruistic anarchism, hedonistic nihilism . . . which excited the undergraduates of 1968 and which until recently were the stock-in-trade of serious journalism' (1992:107). It is this 'spirit of 68' which has prevailed in the 'weakening of the link between sex, procreation, child-care, child-rearing and loyalty in the life-long provision on a non-commercial basis of mutual care within a common place of residence'. It extends to include, without qualification, the 'new generation of feminists, in revolt against "capitalist patriarchy" or "patriarchal capitalism", whether as "feminist Marxists", "material feminists", or "radical feminists"' (1992:61–2) whose 'attack on the family is the last fling of Marxism' (1992:65).

The ease with which these authors dismiss the research and scholarship of critical analysis, including the full range and diversity of feminist critiques, provides a damning indictment of their academic approach, demonstrating a poverty of theory and lack of rigour. Yet their work not only enjoys a significant constituency, appealing to a politically broad church, it is also influential in establishing unexpected alliances. David Green, Director of the right-wing Institute of Economic Affairs, acknowledges the close association of the work of journalists Norman Macrae (*The Sunday Times*) and Melanie Phillips

(*Guardian/Observer*) and the research and writings of Murray, Halsey, Dennis and Erdos, concluding (1992:viii, emphases added):

> The freedom of the press and the courage of a few academics . . . has saved us from monolithic political correctness. The next task is to discover what can be done to restore the ideal of the two-parent family, supported by the grandparents and aunts and uncles of the extended family, and in doing so avoid the extremes, always a possibility when *it becomes necessary to correct fundamentals* (1992:viii).

To resolve the problem of Murray's pathologized communities, the objective is the correction of 'fundamentals'. The focus is those individuals whose actions collectively have destroyed Halsey's 'traditional family system'. According to Green this system is the ideal, and idealized, nuclear family as the kernel of the extended family. Both Murray and the ethical socialists are united in the belief that this system is the primary 'civilising force' within society and all consider that 'dismembered' or 'dysfunctional' families have prevailed because of voluntaristic and avoidable choices made by post-1960s nihilists and hedonists. While judgmentalism is implicit throughout this range of early 1990s work, the affirmation of moral absolutes is its most prevalent feature.

Towards a Rights Agenda for Children and Young People

The abuse, degradation and exclusion of children by adults is a global issue. While guarding against false universalism, the suffering of children at the hands and words of adults is not bounded by class, culture, gender, state or religion. Their enslavement as marginal, easily expendable and unprotected workers in sweatshops, mines, factories and, more recently, highly sophisticated light industry in the world's economic free zones is well-documented. Less thoroughly researched has been the essential contribution made by children and young people in the domestic sphere, as surrogate mothers, cleaners, carers, fetchers and carriers. The street children of Latin American, African and Asian shanty towns are represented in the media as condemnatory evidence of the decivilizing of whole cultures. Stories of child executions at the hands of death squads on the streets of Sao Paulo are matched by disturbing revelations of the sex trade in children in Thailand. The full horror of Rwanda's civil war, like so many others, is transmitted through the experiences of traumatized children who survived as the bereaved witnesses of the terrible slaughter of their loved ones. Undoubtedly, these are matters of profound concern. Their portrayal, however, unacceptably distances media consumers in the West from the depth and complexity of such experiences. Also, it enables those consumers to stand apart from any direct or indirect responsibility for such suffering.

By defining or portraying the experiences of children solely within cultural or societal boundaries, their pain and their exploitation is identified as a domestic issue, yet another expression of ethnic pathology. Yet it is the West, the self-appointed First World, which remorselessly exploits the labour in the sweatshops, the rice fields, the deregulated industrial plants and the mines. It is their affluent men who do business in the vicious and degrading child sex industry. It is the financial dealing of their political leaders and captains of multinational industry which create, without any reciprocal responsibility, the undermining dependency of national debts. At a distance, however, these are worlds apart. Closely associated to economic dominance through dependency is a form of cultural imperialism which implicitly assumes that the children of the First World are protected, cared for and provided for, nurtured, loved and educated, free from poverty, abuse, exploitation, illness and premature death. It is a cruel lie. For, whatever the relative material benefits, quality of life and opportunities self-evident within advanced capitalist societies, structural inequalities, ritualized abuse and the systematic denial of citizen's rights to all under the age of 18 are deeply etched into Britain's social and political landscape.

The Children's Rights Office notes that the United Kingdom is one of the richest nation-states in the world – with its children protected from the fundamental 'difficulties experienced by those in many developing countries of, for example, absolute poverty, malnutrition, death from preventable diseases, bonded child labour and illiteracy' (CRO, 1995a:8). Yet, there are serious problems for children in the UK:

> growing inequality, increased poverty, drug abuse, teenage pregnancy, high levels of violence to children including sexual abuse, growing levels of child prostitution, homelessness, rapidly rising divorce rates, growing problems of suicide and mental illness, a deteriorating environment and alienation from the political process (CRO, 1995a:8).

The preceding chapters have focused on these issues and on the lack of appropriate forums in which children and young people can voice their concerns or participate in their resolution. While politicians, media commentators and academics continue to lay the problems of childhood at the door of the 'disintegrating community' or the 'dismembered family' – arguing, as illustrated in the last section, that the issue is primarily one of moral values – the material realities derived in the determining contexts and structural relations of production (class), reproduction (patriarchy) and neocolonialism ('race') are ignored. The Association of Metropolitan Authorities, in noting that 'children are the most vulnerable group in society', concludes:

> They have no voting rights and therefore no formal avenues to exercise power. They can only experience change through the actions

of adults. Adults in positions of responsibility therefore have a duty to ensure that the rights of children and young people are respected (1995:11).

What this process of adult mediation in all matters means is that ranging from the use of physical punishment in the home, in childcare or in schools, across the board to accessing contraception and abortion advice it is left to adults to decide on the 'best interests' of children in any given situation. As Liberty argues, 'there is a danger that children's rights in areas such as privacy and freedom of information, to name but two, can be randomly violated on the grounds that it is in their best interests' (in NCCL, 1991:69).

Again, the issue tends to be determined primarily on the grounds of moral values and judgments, as illustrated in Chapter 4's discussion of Gillick competence. In this line of moral argument there has been a commitment by adults to 'protecting' children and young people from knowledge and information relevant to their developing sexualities until such a time as adults/professionals/judges consider that they have matured sufficiently to cope with such matters. This returns the discussion to the notion of childhood innocence, effectively a state of ignorance or assumption based on rumour and imagination. It leads to a false prolonging of childhood in which physical and emotional development are allowed to run ahead of appropriate knowledge and understanding. Yet, at the same time in other spheres, children are expected to be rational and all-knowing in identifying the potential consequences of their actions. Nowhere has this been more evident than in the debate over criminal responsibility. Following the decision to prosecute two 10-year-old boys for murder in the case of James Bulger, the aftermath revealed the underlying contradictions implicit in the discourses which contextualize the political management and legal regulation of children. The decision to prosecute flew in the face of the principle, accepted by Parliament in 1969, that there should be no punishment of children without proven moral responsibility and, further, that children should benefit from care and regulation rather than incarceration and punishment. Allan Levy QC, a leading authority on children and the law remains unequivocal in his response to the 'sad message' of the trial of the two boys:

> The full adversarial process of a major criminal prosecution enveloped the two boys . . . The Bulger case has revealed the unacceptable face of our criminal justice system concerning children. It provides an unpalatable insight into outmoded thought, reform denied and the appearance of political calculation (*Guardian*, 29 November 1994).

The final reference, concerning political calculation, was directed against the Home Secretary's intervention to set a minimum-served sentence of 15 years. Gitta Sereny, an authority on the case of Mary Bell (who in 1968 at the age of 10 killed two toddlers) also strongly rejected the 15 year sentence:

It is outrageous, utterly outrageous. What hope do you give them? . . . 15 years for an 11-year-old is the other side of the moon. It is very important for them to be punished for something so wrong but it is not right for all hope to be taken away and for them to be put in a situation in which they cannot but be corrupted (*Guardian*, 8 February 1995).

Apart from the long-term consequences of a sentence eventually leading to young offenders' institutions and adult prisons the issue of equating moral responsibility with age remains critical. In May 1996 an 11-year-old boy was found guilty of manslaughter after he had pushed a concrete block from the top of a nine-storey tower block, killing a 74-year-old woman below. The subsequent trial turned on the issue of whether, in the circumstances, he could distinguish between right and wrong. He was found guilty of manslaughter, which suggests that despite his age the jury considered he could be held fully responsible for his actions. The judge, however, revealed that this conclusion left him with a 'real sentencing problem' (*Guardian*, 14 June 1996) as incarceration would put the boy 'at risk' and seriously inhibit his rehabilitation. Consequently he was given a 3 year supervision order and returned to his family.

Drawing the line of moral responsibility in relation to age and personal development is not straightforward. In May 1996 in Richmond, California, a 6-year-old boy was charged with attempting to unlawfully kill a one-month-old baby. The prosecutor argued that the boy acted with malice aforethought and that it was 'patently obvious' that he 'knew the difference between right and wrong' (*Independent*, 10 May 1996). Jeffrey Butts, of the National Centre for Juvenile Justice, considers that the issue is not restricted simply to the point at which as adults 'we are willing to acknowledge that children don't have the capacity to make good judgments'. More fundamentally, he argues, it extends to preventing 'the rush to take away the status of childhood from children'. This is precisely the point made by Allan Levy in condemning the 'increasingly reactionary approach' in the British criminal justice process which is actually contributing to the 'victimisation of children' (*Guardian*, 29 November 1994). He continues:

The relevance of childhood and children's special need for protection are well recognised in civil law. It is ironic that in circumstances where the fact of childhood needs more, not less, recognition, the agenda often politically motivated, is geared towards equating the child with the fully responsible adult.

Inevitably, what this leads to is the proposition that the 'fact' of childhood, in itself, becomes a mitigating circumstance in the commission of a serious offence. If drawing the line is to be more than an arbitrary endeavour, who draws it and the criteria used to achieve sound and fair judgments are significant issues.

On the one hand, then, there is the denial of children as rational, responsible persons able to receive information, participate in frank and open discussions and come to well-reasoned and appropriately-informed decisions about their interpersonal relationships (family, friends, sexual), about school and about developing sexuality. On the other, there is the imposition, using the full force of the law, of the highest level of rationality and responsibility on children and young people who seriously offend. The paradox is that the same sources appear to propose that childhood represents a period of diminished adult responsibility governing certain actions while being a period of equal responsibility governing others. What is clear from the work of children's advocacy agencies, and from consultation with children and young people, is the lack of any systematic attempt to resolve these contradictions and evolve institutional arrangements which recognize and actively promote the rights of children and young people in accord with the responsibilities placed on them.

As the preceding chapters have concluded, the framework for such arrangements is contained in the UN Convention on the Rights of the Child (United Nations, 1989). The Convention was adopted by the UN General Assembly in 1989 and ratified by the UK Government in December 1991. By 1996 it had received almost universal ratification by the 190 UN member states. The convention comprises over 50 Articles, the main aims of which are to establish the rights of children and young people to adequate and effective care and protection, provide services and facilities appropriate to their fundamental needs and encourage institutional arrangements which enable them to be active participants in their society. The UN Committee expects ratifying states to initiate legal and policy reform and to develop professional agency practices in accordance with the Articles. As an international agreement the Convention is binding in international law. The Articles cover rights and duties across the entire social and community spectrum, providing direction for all state institutionally-based interventionist policies and practices. It recognizes the role and function of the state in supporting parents and carers in the growth, development and socialization of children.

Certain articles frame precise and unambiguous objectives. Article 19, for example, proclaims the right of the child to protection from all forms of physical and mental violence, abuse and neglect. Others, however, are more circumspect but no less significant. Crucial here is Article 3 which states the duty, in all actions, to consider the 'best interests of the child'. Again, the issue of who determines, defines and administers 'best interests' is not so easily identified. If this Article is placed alongside Article 5, which imposes a duty on governments to respect the rights and responsibilities of parents to provide guidance for children 'in line with their evolving capacities', the issue becomes compounded. In England and Wales the 1989 Children Act addressed parental responsibilities in terms of the sum total of 'rights', 'duties', 'power', 'responsibilities' and 'authority' which legally a parent has in relation to its child/children and their property. Most state institutions, childcare professionals and parents/carers would accept that parenthood involves responsibility, if not active decision-making, for the social development and personal guidance of the child. Article 5 underwrites this responsibility, directing states to do the same in providing support, but it is a responsibility left to the discretion of parents or carers as they quantify the 'evolving capacities' of the children in their care. While Article 3 establishes 'best interests' and declares a duty of care and protection there is no formula for establishing 'best interests' in any given circumstance.

The spirit of Articles 5 and 3 does reverse the traditional relationship of parents and carers to children by focusing on some broader conceptualization of 'evolving capacities' and 'best interests'. As the Children's Rights Office states, parents' rights are limited: 'to override the actions of a child only where the child is not competent to understand fully the consequences of their actions, or where failure to intervene would place the child at risk . . .' (CRO, 1995b:12). Much of this, however, carries little weight or relevance while children and young people are excluded and marginalized from the processes, including their status in the family, which govern and determine their lives. How are they to know any different? The Convention proclaims the right to express an opinion and have it taken seriously (Article 12), the right to freedom of expression (Article 13) and the right of access to appropriate information (Article 17). As has been stated elsewhere, 'a balance has to be struck between . . . the child's right to receive information and . . . their right to be protected from material that is likely to be harmful to them' (CRO, 1995b:35). Parents and carers are expected to mediate on these conflicting processes, again reflecting the dichotomy of liberty versus freedom. They become, as they already are, the definers of appropriateness as it relates to their perception of a child's competence. While Article 12 states the right to freedom of expression, legislation does not provide for this within the family, as it is conceived, if not reinforced, as a 'private domain'.

The reservations implicit in the above discussion are not meant to undermine the potential of the UN Convention as a significant forward move for the lives, experiences and decisions of children and young people. Progress can be made, however, only if the ratifying states actively promote, through legislation and policy, the Convention's Articles. Within the UK there is significant complacency linked to a 'little Englander' mentality concerning political sovereignty which has mitigated against the realization of the Convention's objectives. As stated previously, the complacency is derived in the mistaken assumption that the UK already meets most of the key demands made by the Convention and that the Articles are directed elsewhere, towards less 'civilized' societies. The sovereignty issue reflects a deep-seated and mistaken ideology which conflates nationalism, patriotism and xenophobia. It leads to a reluctance to move forward on any initiatives which are seen to be derived outside the narrow confines of the 'British' Parliament and to an explicit rejection of external, progressive, social and political initiatives for change.

Accordingly, in implementing the UN Convention, the UK Government failed 'to undertake a critical self-appraisal of the extent to which UK legislation, policies and practice comply with its principles and standards' (CRO, 1995a:8). Following ratification the UK Government put forward a series of reservations to the UN Secretary General. These focused primarily on immigration, employment and youth justice. In January 1995, following consideration of the UK's initial report, the UN Committee on the Rights of the Child responded by raising 15 substantive issues of concern (CRC, 1995). These included: immigration policy and legislation; coordination of the Convention's implementation; Northern Ireland; healthcare; sex education; physical and sexual abuse; children in care; youth justice, particularly the extension of imprisonment through secure training orders; poverty. One of the most serious issues was that the 'principle of the best interest of the child appears not to be reflected in legislation in such areas as health, education and social security . . .' (1995:3). Further, with regard to schooling, 'the right of the child to express his or her opinion is not solicited' (1995:3). The Committee was 'deeply worried' over 'judicial interpretations of the present law permitting the reasonable chastisement in cases of physical abuse of children within the family context' (1995:4). This led to concern that 'the physical integrity of children' as defined within the Convention was not protected by UK legislative or policy measures. It directed that in terms of 'best interests' and consultation the UK Government should incorporate appropriate and effective measures into rights' policies and legislation. It recommended 'further mechanisms to facilitate the participation of children in decisions affecting them . . .' (1995:5). The force and extent of the UN Committee's response left no doubts as to its dismay at the lack of progress made by the UK Government.

Inevitably, the UK Government 'expressed considerable anger at the explicit criticism of the poor record of the UK in implementing the Convention . . . given the poor record of respecting children which pertains in so many other countries in the world' (CRO, 1995a:8). This brought an immediate rebuke from Thomas Hammerberg, Vice Chair of the UN Committee, who stated that 'of more than 30 governments that have now appeared before the Committee, none has reacted with such hostility as the UK Government to its [the Committee's] observations and recommendations' (CRO, 1995a:8). The UK Government's response typifies a much wider denial of directives, agreements, treaties and conventions initiated and instituted beyond its borders yet demanding monitored, transparent progress within. Again, the politics of sovereignty were easily mobilized and invoked to popularize and represent international agreements as 'destabilizing' or 'interfering' with established, internal state policies and practices. Yet, as argued by the Children's Rights Office (CRO, 1995a:9), the objective of international, binding agreements and their monitoring 'is not to produce a league table of comparative progress' but to consider progress towards agreed aims and given 'resources, political situation, history, stability and culture'. A commitment to such progress, however, cannot be realized through rhetoric. It has to be carried through political will, informed debate and legislative and policy change.

The apparent reluctance of the UK Government to take appropriate action, through legal and policy reform, in implementing the UN Convention does not inspire confidence for the future of a rights agenda in Britain. As this book shows, legal reform and policy initiatives regarding children and young people have been regressive rather than progressive, imbued with characteristic authoritarian principles. The enduring popular imagery continues to promote caricatures of poorly-disciplined children, lawless youth, inadequate parents and failing teachers and social workers. With material realities submerged under wave after wave of adult moral indignation there is little popular constituency for a rights agenda. What has been evident throughout the 1990s is a sustained backlash directed against critical analysis and child-centred policies and practices. While the backlash has been sustained it has failed to eradicate the gradual progress towards a positive rights agenda which aims to secure rights for children and young people independent of but equal in standing to those of adults.

A positive rights agenda has the potential to create conditions necessary for the full and active participation of children and young people. At local, regional and national levels voluntary agencies continue to resist the blend of indifference and hostility directed towards their efforts as advocates and providers. These agencies have been effective, as have some health providers and youth/community services, in promoting the interests and meeting the needs of children. This interventionist and proactive work, along with the resistance of young people themselves, reveals a clear commitment to responding to children as persons rather than as dependants. This includes their active participation in decisions, both in the private and public spheres, which affect their lives. Of particular significance is the quality of life experienced in both family and community contexts.

As children develop, their right to knowledge and information necessarily extends beyond that which is provided within families or through school curricula. While these are the primary sites of their social experiences and socialization they are also institutional settings which limit and confine children's knowledge and understanding. The recent emergence and success of community drop-in centres as providers of informed advice, support and advocacy, governing a range of social, health and economic issues, demonstrates the significance of independent consultation opportunities for children and young people. These processes identify and target children as receivers of information and knowledge through which they can make responsible decisions underpinned by appropriate support. A positive rights agenda also perceives and promotes children as providers of information concerning their social and familial relationships and the administration of their schools, their communities and their physical environment. It challenges the reductionism which has characterized children as no more than passive consumers of community services. In contrast, it promotes full and active participation including effective consultation and monitoring. Until central and local government accept the need to establish children's rights departments which recognize and endorse the unique and developing needs of children and young people, the formal agenda will remain, at best, tokenistic.

The primary obstacles in the path of sound, progressive reform remain the structural relations and social arrangements through which adult power is endured by children. Adult power dominates their personal and social lives and is institutionalized in 'caring' and 'disciplining' agencies alike. As has been evident in the plethora of contemporary scandals, it is a power readily and systematically abused. It is a dangerous and debilitating power, capable of stunting the personal development and potential of even the most resilient children. It is physically and mentally painful, damaging good health and often wreaking havoc in those interpersonal relationships which require love, care and trust. What is so difficult for adults, as the power-brokers, to accept is that the 'crisis' is not one of 'childhood' but one of adultism. In the struggle against the full spectrum of the oppression of children, adults have to address the oppressor within and alongside them. It is imperative that the dominant lie, that adult power and its manifestations are conceived and administered for the benefit of children, is exposed. Equally important is an awareness of the damage done under the guise of protection and through the idealization of 'childhood' and the 'family'. The removal of these obstacles will enable children and young people to experience a more effective, participatory context supported by a positive rights agenda.

Notes on Contributors

Marc Bourhill is a secondary school teacher, with responsibility for special needs, at a Merseyside comprehensive. He is also a Research Associate of the Centre of Studies in Crime and Social Justice at Edge Hill University College. His research interests include: the politics of ageism; deschooling; media constructions of childhood and the processes of demonization.

Vicki Coppock is a Senior Lecturer is Social Policy and Social Work and Staff Associate of the Centre for Studies in Crime and Social Justice at Edge Hill University College. She has extensive professional experience as a psychiatric social worker in both child and adult mental health settings. Her primary teaching and research interests include: mental health; social work and social policy; gender and sexuality; children, young people and social justice. She is co-author (with Deena Haydon and Ingrid Richter) of *The Illusions of Post-Feminism: New Women, Old Myths*, Taylor and Francis, 1995, and is Coordinator of the Young People, Power and Justice Research Group.

Karen Corteen is a full-time postgraduate researcher and sessional tutor in the Centre for Studies in Crime and Social Justice at Edge Hill University College. Her current research is focused primarily on the impact of Section 28 of the Local Government Act and the legal regulation of sex education within schools and youth work. She is co-author (with Deena Haydon) of *Sex Education in Primary Schools: Policy and Practice* (forthcoming). She has considerable youth work experience, particularly working with young women's groups.

Howard Davis is a Researcher at the Centre for Studies in Crime and Social Justice, Edge Hill University College, working on a project (with Phil Scraton) examining institutional responses to survivors and the bereaved in the aftermath of disasters. His research interests include: the consequences of adult abuse of children; bereavement and sudden death; the definition and application of post-traumatic stress disorder. He continues to work part-time as a social worker and has extensive experience in the areas of child protection, HIV/AIDS and bereavement and was a member of Hillsborough Disaster social work team.

Barry Goldson is a Lecturer in the Department of Sociology, Social Policy and Social Work Studies at the University of Liverpool and a Research Associate of the Centre for Studies in Crime and Social Justice, Edge Hill University College. His teaching and research interests include: social policy and social work law; children and young people in public care, youth justice and state institutions; the theoretical and critical analyses of the structural location of children and young people; contemporary children's rights debates. He has many years experience of working directly with children and young people in both the statutory and voluntary sectors and retains a keen interest in youth social work practice.

Deena Haydon is Senior Lecturer in Primary Education at Edge Hill University College and a Staff Research Associate of the Centre for Studies in Crime and Social Justice. She has considerable and diverse experience in primary education and her teaching and research interests include: sex and sexuality education in primary schools; children's rights initiatives and their impact on school policies and practices; the politics of equal opportunities in education; contemporary critical debates in educational policy and practice. She is co-author of *The Illusions of Post-Feminism: New Women, Old Myths*, Taylor and Francis, 1995 (with Vicki Coppock and Ingrid Richter), of *Getting Personal*, PSE Scheme for Primary Schools, Folens, 1996 (with Pat King and Chris Moorcroft) and of *Sex Education in Primary Schools: Policy and Practice*, forthcoming (with Karen Corteen).

Phil Scraton is Professor of Criminology and Criminal Justice and Director of the Centre for Studies in Crime and Social Justice at Edge Hill University College. With Kathryn Chadwick he runs the Centre's postgraduate research and Masters' programmes. His primary research interests include: the politics and regulation of sexuality; the rights of survivors and the bereaved in the aftermath of disasters; police powers and accountability; deaths in custody; critical analysis and its application. He is author of *The State of the Police*, Pluto, 1985, and editor of *Law, Order and the Authoritarian State*, Open University Press, 1987. He is co-author of *In the Arms of the Law*, Pluto, 1987 (with Kathryn Chadwick), *Prisons Under Protest*, Open University Press, 1991 (with Joe Sim and Paula Skidmore), and *No Last Rights: The Denial of Justice and the Promotion of Myth in the Aftermath of the Hillsborough Disaster*, LCC/Alden Press, 1995 (with Ann Jemphrey and Sheila Coleman). He has written extensively on a range of human rights and social justice issues.

All contributors are members of the Young People, Power and Justice Research Group, Centre for Studies in Crime and Social Justice, Edge Hill University College, Ormskirk, Lancashire L39 4QP.

References

ABBOTT, P. and WALLACE, C. (1992) *The Family and the New Right*, London, Pluto Press.

ADAMS, P., BERG, L., BERGER, N., DUANE, M., NEILL, A. S. and OLLENDORFF, R. (1972) *Children's Rights*, London, Elek Books.

AINLEY, P. (1988) *From School to YTS: Education and Training in England and Wales, 1944–1987*, Milton Keynes, Open University Press.

ALANEN, L. (1994) 'Gender and generation: Feminism and the 'child question', in QVORTRUP, J. *et al.* (Eds) *Childhood Matters: Social Theory, Practice and Politics*, Aldershot, Avebury.

ALLEN, R. (1991) 'Out of jail: The reduction in the use of penal custody for male juveniles 1981–88', *Howard Journal of Criminal Justice*, **30**, pp. 30–52.

ANDERSON, D. and DAWSON, G. (Eds) (1986) *Family Portaits*, London, Social Affairs Unit.

ANDERSON, M. (1983) 'How much has the family changed?', *New Society*, 27 October.

ANDERSON, M. (1995) *Today's Families in Historical Context*, Paper to Church of England/Joseph Rowntree Foundation Seminar.

ARCHARD, D. (1993) *Children's Rights and Childhood*, London, Routledge.

ARIÈS, P. (1962) *Centuries of Childhood*, Harmondsworth, Penguin.

ARMSTRONG, D. (1983) *The Political Anatomy of the Body*, Cambridge, Cambridge University Press.

ASHTON, D., MAGUIRE, M. and SPILSBURY, M. (1990) *Restructuring the Labour Market: The Implications for Youth*, London, Macmillan.

ASSOCIATION OF METROPOLITAN AUTHORITIES (1993) *Funding of Grant-Maintained Schools*, Briefing Paper, 13 May, London, Association of Metropolitan Authorities.

ASSOCIATION OF METROPOLITAN AUTHORITIES (1995) *Checklist for Children: Local Authorities and the UN Convention on the Rights of the Child*, London, AMA/CRO.

BAINHAM, A. (1989) *Parents, Children and the State*, London, Sweet & Maxwell.

BALL, S. J. (1990) *Politics and Policy Making in Education: Explorations in Policy Sociology*, London, Routledge.

References

BARDY, M. (1994) 'The manuscript of the 100-years project: Towards a revision', in QVORTRUP, J. *et al.* (Eds) *Childhood Matters: Social Theory, Practice and Politics*, Aldershot, Avebury.

BARRETT, M. (1980) *Women's Oppression Today*, London, Verso.

BARRETT, M. and MCINTOSH, M. (1982) *The Anti-Social Family*, London, Verso.

BARTON, L. and MEIGHAN, R. (Eds) (1978) *Sociological Interpretations of Schooling and Classrooms: A Reappraisal*, Nafferton, Nafferton Books.

BARTON, L. and MEIGHAN, R. (Eds) (1979) *Schools, Pupils and Deviance*, Nafferton, Nafferton Books.

BASH, L. and COULBY, D. (1989) *The Education Reform Act: Competition and Control*, London, Cassell.

BATES, I., CLARKE, J., COHEN, P., FINN, D., MOORE, R. and WILLIS, P. (1984) *Schooling for the Dole? The New Vocationalism*, London, Macmillan.

BATES, I. and RISEBOROUGH, G. (1993) *Youth and Inequality*, Buckingham, Open University Press.

BATES, P. (1994) 'Children in secure psychiatric units: Re K, W and H – "Out of sight, out of mind"?', *Journal of Child Law*, **6** (3), pp. 131–7.

BEAN, P. and MELVILLE, J. (1989) *Lost Children of the Empire*, London, Hyman.

BEBBINGTON, A. and MILES, J. (1989) 'The background of children who enter local authority care', *British Journal of Social Work*, **19**, pp. 349–68.

BELL, C. and ROBERTS, H. (1984) *Social Researching: Politics, Problems, Practice*, London, Routledge and Kegan Paul.

BELL, S. (1988) *When Salem Came to the Boro: The True Story of the Cleveland Child Abuse Crisis*, London, Pan Paperbacks.

BEN, C. and CHITTY, C. (1995) *Thirty Years On: Is Comprehensive Education Alive and Well, or Struggling to Survive?*, London, Fulton.

BERESFORD, S. (1994) 'Lesbians in residence and parental responsibility cases', *Family Law*, November, pp. 643–5.

BERG, I. (1973) *Education and Jobs: The Great Training Robbery*, London, Penguin.

BERNSTEIN, B. (Ed.) (1972) *Class, Codes and Control*, London, Routledge and Kegan Paul.

BEVERIDGE, W. (1942) *Social Insurance and Allied Services*, Cmnd 6404, London, HMSO.

BLACKMORE, J. (1984) 'Delinquency theory and practice: A link through IT', *Youth and Policy*, **9**.

BOARD OF EDUCATION (1926) *Report of the Consultative Committee on the Education of the Adolescent (First Hadow Report)*, London, HMSO.

BOARD OF EDUCATION (1931) *Report of the Consultative Committee on the Primary School (Second Hadow Report)*, London, HMSO.

BOARD OF EDUCATION (1933) *Report of the Consultative Committee on Infant and Nursery Schools (Third Hadow Report)*, London HMSO.

BOARD OF EDUCATION (1938) *Report of the Consultative Committee on Secondary Education with Special Reference to Grammar Schools (The Spens Report)*, London, HMSO.

BOARD OF EDUCATION (1943a) *Report of the Committee of the Secondary School Examinations Council on Curriculum and Examinations in Secondary Schools (The Norwood Report)*, London, HMSO.

BOARD OF EDUCATION (1943b) *Educational Reconstruction* (White Paper), Cmnd 6458, London, HMSO.

BOTTOMS, A. (1995) *Intensive Community Supervision of Young Offenders: Outcomes, Process and Cost*, Cambridge, University of Cambridge Institute of Criminology.

BOTTOMLEY COMMITTEE (1988) *The Line of Least Resistance: The Report of the Children's Society's Advisory Committee on Penal Custody and Its Alternatives for Juveniles*, London, The Children's Society.

BOWE, R., BALL, S. and GOLD, A. (1992) *Reforming Education and Changing Schools: Case Studies in Policy Sociology*, London, Routledge.

BOWLBY, J. (1951) *Maternal Care and Mental Health*, Geneva, WHO.

BOWLBY, J. (1953) *Child Care and the Growth of Love*, Harmondsworth, Penguin.

BOWLBY, J. (1988) *A Secure Base: Clinical Applications of Attachment Theory*, Bristol, Arrowsmith.

BOWLES, B. and GINTIS, H. (1976) *Schooling in Capitalist America: Educational Reform and the Contradictions of Economic Life*, London, Routledge and Kegan Paul.

BOX, S. (1981) *Deviance, Reality and Society*, London: Holt, Rinehart & Winston.

BRIDENTHAL, R. (1982) 'The family: The view from a room of her own', in THORNE, B. and YALLOM, M. (Eds) *Rethinking the Family: Some Feminist Questions*, Harlow, Longman.

BRITISH YOUTH COUNCIL (1992) *The Time of Their Lives*, London, BYC.

BROWN, P. (1987) *Schooling Ordinary Kids*, London, Routledge.

BROWN, P. (1990) 'Schooling and economic life in the UK', in CHISHOLM L. (Ed.) *Childhood, Youth and Social Change: A Comparative Perspective*, London, Falmer Press.

BROWNMILLER, S. (1976) *Against Our Will: Men, Women and Rape*, Harmondsworth, Penguin.

BURGHES, L. (1994) *Lone Parenthood and Family Disruption: The Outcomes for Children*, London, Family Policy Studies Centre.

BURMAN, E. (1994) *Deconstructing Developmental Psychology*, London, Routledge.

BUTLER-SLOSS, E. (1988) *Report of the Inquiry into Child Abuse in Cleveland, 1987*, Cmnd 412, London, HMSO.

CAIN, M. (Ed.) (1989) *Growing Up Good: Policing the Behaviour of Girls in Europe*, London, Sage.

CALOUSTE GULBENKIAN FOUNDATION (1993) *One Scandal Too Many . . . the*

Case for Comprehensive Protection for Children in all Settings, London, Calouste Gulbenkian Foundation.

CAMPBELL, A. (1981) *Girl Delinquents*, Oxford, Blackwell.

CAMPBELL, B. (1988) *Unofficial Secrets: Child Sexual Abuse: The Cleveland Case*, London, Virago.

CAMPBELL, B. (1993) *Goliath: Britain's Dangerous Places*, London, Methuen.

CAMPBELL, B. (1995) 'Hard lessons', *Diva*, August, pp. 18–20.

CANNAN, C. (1992) *Changing Families, Changing Welfare*, Hemel Hempstead, Harvester Wheatsheaf.

CARLEN, P., GLEESON, D. and WARDHAUGH, J. (1992) *Truancy: The Politics of Compulsory Schooling*, Buckingham, Open University Press.

CARPENTER, M. (1851) *Reformatory Schools for the Children of the Perishing and Dangerous Classes and for Juvenile Offenders*, London, Gilpin.

CARPENTER, M. (1853) *Juvenile Delinquents, Their Condition and Treatment*, London, Cash.

CENTRAL ADVISORY COUNCIL FOR EDUCATION (ENGLAND) (1954) *Early Leaving*, London, HMSO.

CENTRAL ADVISORY COUNCIL FOR EDUCATION (ENGLAND) (1959) *15 to 18, Volume One: Report (The Crowther Report)*, London, HMSO.

CENTRAL ADVISORY COUNCIL FOR EDUCATION (ENGLAND) (1963) *Half Our Future (The Newsom Report)*, London, HMSO.

CENTRE FOR CONTEMPORARY CULTURAL STUDIES (1981) *Unpopular Education: Schooling and Social Democracy in England since 1944*, London, Hutchinson.

CHIBNALL, S. (1977) *Law and Order News*, London, Tavistock.

CHILDREN'S LEGAL CENTRE (1991) 'Young people, mental health and the law', *Childright*, **78**, pp. 23–5.

CHILDREN'S LEGAL CENTRE (1993) 'Mental health code revised', *Childright*, **101**, pp. 7–8.

CHILDREN'S LEGAL CENTRE (1994) 'How schools exclude black children', *Childright*, **109**, September, pp. 13–14.

CHILDREN'S LEGAL CENTRE (1995) 'Consent to medical treatment – young people's legal rights', *Childright*, **115**, April, pp. 11–14.

CHILDREN'S RIGHTS DEVELOPMENT UNIT (CRDU) (1994) *UK Agenda for Children*, London, CRDU.

CHILDREN'S SOCIETY ADVISORY COMMITTEE ON JUVENILE CUSTODY AND ITS ALTERNATIVES (1993) *A False Sense of Security: The Case Against Locking Up More Children*, London, The Children's Society.

CHISHOLM, L. (1990) 'A sharper lens or a new camera? Youth research, young people and social change in Britain', in CHISHOLM, L. *et al.* (Eds) *Childhood, Youth and Social Change: A Comparative Perspective*, London, Falmer Press.

CHITTY, C. (1989) *Towards a New Education System: The Victory of the New Right*, London, Falmer Press.

CHITTY, C. (1992) *The Education System Transformed*, Chorlton, Baseline Books.

CHITTY, C. and SIMON, B. (Eds) (1993) *Education Answers Back: Critical Responses to Government Policy*, London, Lawrence & Wishart.

CHOMSKY, N. (1989) *Necessary Illusions: Thought Control in Democratic Societies*, London, Pluto.

CLARK, D. (1994) 'Roundabouts and swings – recent court decisions about the representation of older children', *Panel News*, **7** (4), December, pp. 27–33.

CLARKE, J. (Ed.) (1993) *A Crisis in Care? Challenges to Social Work*, London, Sage/Open University.

CLEVELAND REFUGE AND AID FOR WOMEN AND CHILDREN (1984) *Private Violence: Public Shame*, Middlesborough, CRAWC.

COCKBURN, C. (1987) *Two-Track Training: Sex Inequalities and the YTS*, Basingstoke, Macmillan.

COHEN, S. (1973) *Folk Devils and Moral Panics: The Creation of Mods and Rockers*, London, Paladin.

COHEN, S. (1983) 'Social control talk: Telling stories about correctional change', in GARLAND, D. and YOUNG, P. (Eds) *The Power to Punish: Contemporary Penality and Social Analysis*, London, Heinemann.

COHEN, S. (1985) *Visions of Social Control: Crime, Punishment and Classification*, London, Polity Press.

COHEN, S. (1987) *Folk Devils and Moral Panics: The Creation of the Mods and Rockers* (3rd Edn), Oxford, Blackwell.

COHEN, S. and YOUNG, J. (Eds) (1973) *The Manufacture of News: Deviance, Social Problems and the Mass Media*, London, Constable.

COLEMAN, S., JEMPHREY, A., SCRATON, P. and SKIDMORE, P. (1990) *Hillsborough and After: The Liverpool Experience: First Report of The Hillsborough Project*, Liverpool, Liverpool City Council.

COLES, B. (1995) *Youth and Social Policy: Youth Citizenship and Young Careers*, London, University College London Press Limited.

COLVIN, M. (1989) *Section 28: A Practical Guide to the Law and Its Implications*, London, National Council for Civil Liberties.

COMMISSION FOR RACIAL EQUALITY (1992) *Submission from the Commission for Racial Equality to the Royal Commission on Criminal Justice*, London, CRE.

COMMITTEE ON HIGHER EDUCATION (1963) *Higher Education: Report (The Robbins Report)*, Cmnd 2154, London, HMSO.

COMMUNITY RELATIONS COMMISSION (1974) *The Educational Needs of Children from Minority Groups*, London, CRC.

CONNELL, B., RADICAN, N. and MARTIN, P. (1987) *The Changing Faces of Masculinity*, Sydney, Macquarie University Press.

COOPER, D. (1989) 'Positive images in Haringey: A struggle for identity', in JONES, C. and MAHONY, P. (Eds) *Learning Our Lines: Sexuality and Social Control in Education*, London, The Women's Press.

References

COOTE, A., HARMAN, H. and HEWITT, P. (1990) *The Family Way: A New Approach to Policy-Making*, London, Institute of Public Policy Research.

COOTER, R. (Ed.) (1992) *In the Name of the Child: Health and Welfare, 1880–1940*, London, Routledge.

COPPOCK, V., HAYDON, D. and RICHTER, I. (1995) *The Illusions of 'Post-Feminism': New Women, Old Myths*, London, Taylor and Francis.

CORSON, D. (Ed.) (1991) *Education for Work: Background to Policy and Curriculum*, Clevedon, Multilingual Matters.

COSIN, B. R., DALE, I. R., ESLAND, G. M., MacKINNON, D. and SWIFT, D. F. (1971) *School and Society: A Sociological Reader*, London, Routledge and Kegan Paul.

COSIS-BROWN, H. (1991) 'Competent child-focused practice; Working with lesbian and gay carers', *Adoption and Fostering*, **15** (2).

COWARD, R. (1983) *Patriarchal Precedents*, London, Routledge and Kegan Paul.

COX, C. B. and BOYSON, R. (Eds) (1975) *Black Paper 1975: The Fight for Education*, London, J.M. Dent.

COX, C. B. and DYSON, A. E. (Eds) (1969a) *Fight for Education: Black Paper One*, London, Critical Quarterly Society.

COX, C. B. and DYSON, A. E. (Eds) (1969b) *The Crisis in Education: Black Paper Two*, London, Critical Quarterly Society.

COX, C. B. and DYSON, A. E. (Eds) (1971) *Goodbye Mr Short: Black Paper Three*, London, Critical Quarterly Society.

CRC (1995) Consideration of Reports Submitted by States Parties under Article 44 of the Convention: Concluding observations of the CRC: UK and Northern Ireland Committee on the Rights of the Child 8th Session, 27 January 1995.

CREAM, J. (1993) 'Child sexual abuse and the symbolic geographies of Cleveland', *Society and Space*, **II**.

CRISP, A. (1994) 'Children first', *Community Care*, 28 July–3 August, pp. 2–3.

CRISP, A. (1995) 'The social context of youth crime', *AJJUST NOW*, **36**, pp. 13–15.

CRO (1995a) *Making the Convention Work for Children*, London, Children's Rights Office.

CRO (1995b) *Building Small Democracies*, London, Children's Rights Office.

DALE, R. (Ed.) (1985) *Education, Training and Employment: Towards a New Vocationalism?*, Oxford, Pergamon.

DALE, R., ESLAND, G. and MacDONALD, M. (Eds) (1976) *Schooling and Capitalism: A Sociological Reader*, London, Routledge and Kegan Paul.

DALE, R., ESLAND, G., FERGUSON, R. and MacDONALD, M. (Eds) (1981) *Education and the State, Vol 1: Schooling and the National Interest*, London, Falmer Press.

DALLOS, R. and McLAUGHLIN, E. (Eds) (1993) *Social Problems and the Family*, London, Sage/Open University.

DAVID, M. E. (1986) 'Moral and maternal: The family in the New Right', in LEVITAS, R. (Ed.) *The Ideology of the New Right*, Cambridge, Polity Press.

DAVID, M. E. (1993) 'Theories of family change, motherhood and education', in ARNOT, M. and WEILER, K. (Eds) *Feminism and Social Justice in Education*, London, Falmer Press.

DAVIE, R. and GALLOWAY, D. (Eds) (1996) *Listening to Children in Education*, London, Fulton.

DAVIES, J. (Ed.) (1993) *The Family: Is It Just Another Lifestyle Choice?*, London, Institute of Economic Affairs.

DAVIS, K. (1948) *Human Society*, New York, Macmillan.

DELAMONT, S. (1976) *Interaction in the Classroom*, London, Methuen.

DELAMONT, S. (1983) *Interaction in the Classroom* 2nd Edition, London, Methuen.

DELAMONT, S. (Ed.) (1984) *Readings on Interaction in the Classroom*, London, Methuen.

DELPHY, C. (1976) 'Continuities and discontinuities in marriage and divorce', in BARKER, D. and ALLEN, S. (Eds) *Sexual Divisions and Society*, London, Tavistock.

DELPHY, C. and LEONARD, D. (1992) *Familiar Exploitation: A New Analysis of Marriage in Contemporary Western Societies*, Cambridge, Polity Press.

DE MAUSE, L. (1976) *The History of Childhood: The Evolution of Parent-Child Relationships as a Factor in History*, London, Souvenir Press.

DENNIS, N. (1993) *Rising Crime and the Dismembered Family: How Conformist Intellectuals Have Campaigned Against Common Sense*, London, Institute of Economic Affairs.

DENNIS, N. and ERDOS, G. (1992) *Families Without Fatherhood*, London, Institute of Economic Affairs.

DENNIS, N., HENRIQUES, F. and SLAUGHTER, C. (1956) *Coal Is Our Life*, London, Eyre & Spottiswoode.

DEPARTMENT FOR EDUCATION (1994) *Bullying: Don't Suffer in Silence. An Anti-Bullying Pack for Schools*, London, HMSO.

DEPARTMENT OF CULTURAL STUDIES (1991) *Education Limited: Schooling, Training and the New Right in England Since 1979*, London, Unwin Hyman.

DEPARTMENT OF EDUCATION AND SCIENCE (1965) 'The Organisation of Secondary Education', Circular 10/65, London, HMSO.

DEPARTMENT OF EDUCATION AND SCIENCE (1967) *Children and Their Primary Schools: Volume One, Report (The Plowden Report)*, London, HMSO.

DEPARTMENT OF EDUCATION AND SCIENCE (1977) *Education in Schools: A Consultative Document*, Cmnd 6869, London, HMSO.

DEPARTMENT OF EDUCATION AND SCIENCE (1985) *Better Schools*, Cmnd 9469, London, HMSO.

DEPARTMENT OF EDUCATION AND SCIENCE (1987) 'Sex education at school', Circular No 11/87, 25 September, London, HMSO.

DEPARTMENT OF EDUCATION AND SCIENCE (1989) *Discipline in Schools: Report of the Committee of Enquiry Chaired by Lord Elton*, London, HMSO.

DEPARTMENT OF HEALTH (1986) *NHS Psychiatric Admissions in England*, London, HMSO.

DEPARTMENT OF HEALTH (1992) *Choosing with Care: Report of the Committee of Inquiry into the Selection, Development and Management of Staff in Children's Homes*, London, HMSO.

DEPARTMENT OF HEALTH (1994) *The UN Convention on the Rights of the Child: The UK's First Report to the UN Committee on the Rights of the Child*, London, HMSO.

DEPARTMENT OF HEALTH AND WELSH OFFICE (1993) *Code of Practice: Mental Health Act 1983*, London, HMSO.

DEPARTMENT OF HEALTH AND DEPARTMENT FOR EDUCATION (1995) *A Handbook on Child and Adolescent Mental Health*, London, HMSO.

DEPARTMENT OF SOCIAL SECURITY (1993) *Households Below Average Income*, London, HMSO.

DEWS, V. and WATTS, J. (1994) *Review of Probation Officer Recruitment and Qualifying Training*, London, Home Office.

DFE (1994) 'Sex Education in Schools', Circular 5/94, London, Department for Education.

DOBASH, R. E. and DOBASH, R. (1980) *Violence Against Wives: A Case Against the Patriarchy*, London, Open Books.

DOBASH, R. E. and DOBASH, R. (1992) *Women, Violence and Social Change*, London, Routledge.

DOMINELLI, L. (1988) *Anti-Racist Social Work*, London, Macmillan.

DOMINELLI, L. and McLEOD, E. (1989) *Feminist Social Work*, London, Macmillan.

DONZELOT, J. (1980) *The Policing of Families*, London, Hutchinson.

DRAKEFORD, M. (1995) 'The Social Context of Youth Justice', *AJJUST NOW*, **36**, pp. 10–12.

DURHAM, M. (1991) *Sex and Politics: The Family and Morality in the Thatcher Years*, London, Macmillan.

EDELMAN, M. (1977) *Political Language: Words that Succeed and Policies that Fail*, New York, Academic Press.

EDHOLM, F. (1991) 'The unnatural family', in LONEY, M., BOCOCK, R., CLARKE, J., COCHRANE, A., GRAHAM, P. and WILSON, M. (Eds) *The State or the Market: Politics and Welfare in Contemporary Britain*, London, Sage/ Open University.

EDWARDS, S. (1989) *Policing 'Domestic' Violence*, London, Sage.

EEKELAAR, J. and DINGWALL, R. (1990) *The Reform of Child Care Law: A Practical Guide to the Children Act 1989*, London, Routledge.

EGGLESTON, J. (1977) *The Sociology of the School Curriculum*, London, Routledge and Kegan Paul.

EICHLER, M. (1981) 'The inadequacy of the monolithic model of the family', *Canadian Journal of Sociology*, **6**.

ELLIOT, D. (1988) *Gender, Delinquency and Society*, Avebury, Gower.

EMSLEY, C. (1987) *Crime and Society in England, 1750–1900*, London, Longman.

ENGELBERT, A. (1994) 'Words of childhood: Differentiated but different. Implications for social policy', in QVORTRUP, J. *et al.* (Eds) *Childhood Matters, Social Theory, Practice and Politics*, Aldershot, Avebury.

ENGELS, F. (1968) *The Condition of the Working Class in England*, St Albans, Granada Publishing.

ENGLER, S. (1990) 'Illusory equality: The discipline-based anticipatory socialization of university students', in CHISHOLM, L. *et al.* (Eds) *Childhood, Youth and Social Change: A Comparative Perspective*, London, Falmer Press.

ENNEW, J. (1994) 'Time for children time for adults', in QVORTRUP, J. *et al.* (Eds) *Childhood Matters: Social Theory, Practice and Politics*, Aldershot, Avebury.

EPSTEIN, D. and JOHNSON, R. (1994) 'On the straight and narrow: The heterosexual presumption, homophobia and schools', in EPSTEIN, D. (Ed.) *Challenging Lesbian and Gay Inequalities in Education*, Buckingham, Open University Press.

EVANS, D. (1994) 'Fallen angels? The material construction of children as sexual citizens', *International Journal of Children's Rights*, **2**, pp. 1–33.

EVANS, D. (1995) '(Homo)sexual citizenship: A queer kind of justice', in WILSON, A. R. (Ed.), *A Simple Matter of Justice?*, London, Cassell.

EVANS, D. T. (1989) 'Section 28: Law, myth and paradox', *Critical Social Policy*, **27**, Winter, pp. 73–95.

EVETTS, J. (1973) *The Sociology of Educational Ideas*, London, Routledge and Kegan Paul.

FARSON, R. (1974) *Birthrights*, New York, Macmillan.

FEMINIST REVIEW COLLECTIVE (1988) *Family Secrets: Child Sexual Abuse*, Special Issue, **28**.

FENNELL, P. (1992) 'Informal compulsion: The psychiatric treatment of juveniles under common law', *Journal of Social Welfare and Family Law*, **4**, pp. 311–13.

FERGUSON, A. (1989) *Blood at the Root: Motherhood, Sexuality and Male Dominance*, London, Pandora Press.

FERNANDO, S. (1991) *Mental Health, Race and Culture*, London, Macmillan.

FERNANDO, S. (1995) *Mental Health in a Multi-Ethnic Society*, London, Routledge.

FERRI, E. (1993) *Life at 33: The Fifth Follow-Up of the National Child Development Study*, London, National Children's Bureau.

FIDDY, R. (1984) 'YOP, that's youth off pavements innit', in SCHOSTAK, J. F. and COGAN, T. (Eds) *Pupil Experience*, Beckenham, Croom Helm.

FINCH, J. (1984) 'It's great to have someone to talk to: The ethics and politics of interviewing women', in STANLEY, L. and WISE, S., *Breaking Out:*

Feminist Consciousness and Feminist Research, London, Routledge and Kegan Paul.

FINCH, J. (1989) *Family Obligations and Social Change*, Cambridge, Polity Press.

FINCH, J. and GROVES, D. (Eds) (1983) *A Labour of Love*, London, Routledge.

FINCH, J. and MASON, J. (1992) *Negotiating Family Responsibilities*, London, Routledge.

FINKELHOR, D. (1986) *A Source Book on Child Sexual Abuse*, London, Sage.

FIRESTONE, S. (1972) *The Dialectic of Sex*, London, Paladin.

FLUDE, M. and AHIER, J. (Eds) (1974) *Educability, Schools and Ideology*, London, Croom Helm.

FORD, J., MONGON, D. and WHELAN, M. (1982) *Special Education and Social Control: Invisible Disasters*, London, Routledge and Kegan Paul.

FOUCAULT, M. (1977) *Discipline and Punish: The Birth of the Prison*, London, Allen & Unwin.

FOUCAULT, M. (1979) 'On governmentality', *Ideology and Consciousness*, **6**, pp. 5–21.

FOUCAULT, M. (1980) 'Loving children', *Semiotext(e)*, Special Intervention Series 2, Summer.

FOX-HARDING, L. (1996) *Family, State and Social Policy*, London, Macmillan.

FRANKLIN, B. (Ed.) (1986) *The Rights of Children*, London, Basil Blackwell.

FRANKLIN, B. and PARTON, N. (1991) 'Media reporting of social work: A framework for analysis', in FRANKLIN, B. and PARTON, N. (Eds) *Social Work, the Media and Public Relations*, London, Routledge and Kegan Paul.

FREEMAN, M. D. A. (1983) *The Rights and Wrongs of Children*, London, Frances Pinter.

FREEMAN, M. D. A. (1993) 'Removing rights from adolescents', *Adoption and Fostering*, **17** (1), pp. 14–21.

FREIRE, P. (1972) *Pedagogy of the Oppressed*, Harmondsworth, Penguin.

FROST, N. (1990) 'Official intervention and child protection: The relationship between state and family in contemporary Britain', in THE VIOLENCE AGAINST CHILDREN STUDY GROUP, *Taking Child Abuse Seriously*, London, Unwin Hyman.

FROST, N. and STEIN, M. (1989) *The Politics of Child Welfare*, London, Harvester Wheatsheaf.

FROST, N. and STEIN, M. (1992) 'Empowerment and child welfare', in COLEMAN, J. C. and WARREN-ADAMSON, C. (Eds) *Youth Policy in the 1990s: The Way Forward*, London, Routledge.

GAMBLE, A. (1981) *Britain in Decline*, London, Macmillan.

GAMBLE, A. and WALTON, P. (1976) *Capitalism in Crisis: Inflation and the State*, London, Macmillan.

GARLAND, D. and YOUNG, P. (Eds) (1983) *The Power to Punish: Contemporary Penality and Social Analysis*, London, Heinemann.

GELIS, J. (1986) 'The evolution of the status of the child in western Europe', *Social Research*, **53** (4), Winter.

GELLES, R. J. and CORNELL, C. P. (1990) *Intimate Violence in Families*, London, Sage.

GENDERS, E. and PLAYER, E. (1989) *Race Relations in Prisons*, Oxford, Clarendon Press.

GIBSON, B. (1995) 'Young people, bad news, enduring principles', *Youth and Policy*, **48**, pp. 64–70.

GILLIS, J. (1974) *Youth and History*, London, Academic Press.

GILROY, P. (1987) 'The myth of black criminality', in SCRATON, P. (Ed.) *Law, Order and the Authoritarian State*, Milton Keynes, Open University Press.

GITTINS, D. (1985) *The Family in Question: Challenging Households and Familial Ideologies*, London, Macmillan.

GLASGOW MEDIA GROUP (1976) *Bad News*, London, Routledge and Kegan Paul.

GLASGOW MEDIA GROUP (1980) *More Bad News*, London, Routledge and Kegan Paul.

GLASGOW MEDIA GROUP (1982) *Really Bad News*, London, Routledge and Kegan Paul.

GLENDINNING, C. and MILLAR, J. (Eds) (1987) *Women and Poverty in Britain*, London, Harvester Wheatsheaf.

GOLDING, P. (1991) 'Do-gooders on display: Social work, public attitudes, and the mass media', in FRANKLIN, B. and PARTON, N. (Eds) *Social Work, the Media and Public Relations*, London, Routledge and Kegan Paul.

GOLDING, P. and MIDDLETON, S. (1979) 'Making claims; News media and the welfare state', *Media, Culture and Society*, **1**, pp. 5–21.

GOLDING, W. (1959) *Lord of the Flies*, New York, Capricorn.

GOLDMAN, R. and GOLDMAN, J. (1982) *Children's Sexual Thinking*, London, Routledge and Kegan Paul.

GOLDSON, B. (1994) 'The changing face of youth justice', *Childright*, **105**, April, pp. 5–6.

GOLDTHORPE, J. H., LOCKWOOD, D., BECHOFER, F. and PLATT, J. (1969) *The Affluent Worker in the Class Structure*, Cambridge, Cambridge University Press.

GOODMAN, P. (1971) *Compulsory Miseducation*, Harmondsworth, Penguin.

GORDON, C. (Ed.) (1980) *Michel Foucault: Power, Knowledge, Selected Interviews and Other Writings, 1972–1977*, Brighton, Harvester Press.

GORDON, L. (1982) 'Why nineteenth-century feminists did not support "birth control" and twentieth-century feminists do: Feminism, reproduction and the family', in THORNE, B. and YALLOM, M. (Eds) *Rethinking the Family: Some Feminist Questions*, Harlow, Longman.

GORDON, L. (1989) *Heroes of Their Own Lives: The Politics and History of Family Violence*, London, Virago.

GORDON, P. (1983) *White Law: Racism in the Police, Courts and Prisons*, London, Pluto Press.

References

GOUGH, I. (1979) *The Political Economy of the Welfare State*, London, Macmillan.

GOULD, J. (1977) *The Attack on Higher Education: Marxist and Radical Penetration*, London, Institute for the Study of Conflict.

GOVERNMENT CENTRAL STATISTICAL OFFICE (1994) *Social Focus on Children 1994*, London, HMSO.

GRAEF, R. (1995) 'Media and political interest in youth crime in the UK', in THE HOWARD LEAGUE, *Child Offenders: UK and International Practice*, London, Howard League.

GRAHAM, H. (1984) *Women, Health and the Family*, London, Harvester Wheatsheaf.

GRIFFIN, C. (1985) *Typical Girls? Young Women from School to the Job Market*, London, Routledge and Kegan Paul.

GRIFFIN, C. (1993) *Representations of Youth: The Study of Youth and Adolescence in Britain and America*, Cambridge, Polity Press.

GRIFFIN, S. (1993) 'Fear of a black (and working-class) planet: Young women and the racialization of reproductive politics', in WILKINSON, S. and KITZINGER, C. (Eds) *Heterosexuality: A Feminism and Psychology Reader*, London, Sage.

GRIMSHAW, R. and BERRIDGE, D. (1994) *Educating Disruptive Children: Placement and Progress in Residential Special Schools for Pupils with Emotional and Behavioural Difficulties*, London, National Children's Bureau.

GRIMSHAW, R. and SUMNER, M. (1991) *What's Happening to Childcare Assessment?*, London, National Children's Bureau.

GURA, P. (1994) 'Childhood: A multiple reality', in *Early Child Development and Care*, **98**, Gordon and Breach Science Publishers, pp. 97–111.

HAFFNER, D. W. (1992) 'Sexuality education in policy and practice: Foreword', in SEARS, J. T. (Ed.) *Sexuality and the Curriculum: The Politics and Practices of Sexuality Education*, New York, NY Teachers College, Columbia University.

HAGELL, A. and NEWBURN, T. (1994) *Persistent Young Offenders*, London, Policy Studies Institute.

HALL, L. and LLOYD, S. (1993) *Surviving Child Sexual Abuse*, 2nd Edn, London, Falmer Press.

HALL, S. (1973) 'A world at one with itself', in COHEN, S. and YOUNG, J. (Eds) *The Manufacture of News: Social Problems, Deviance and the Mass Media*, London, Constable.

HALL, S. (1979) 'The great moving right show', *Marxism Today*, January, pp. 14–19.

HALL, S. (1995) 'Grasping at straws: The idealisation of the material in liberal conceptions of youth crime', *Youth and Policy*, **48**, Spring, pp. 49–63.

HALL, S., CRITCHER, C., JEFFERSON, T., CLARKE, J. and ROBERTS, B. (1978) *Policing the Crisis: Mugging, the State and Law and Order*, Basingstoke, Macmillan.

HAMMERSLEY, M. and WOODS, P. (Eds) (1984) *Life in School: The Sociology of Pupil Culture*, Milton Keynes, Open University Press.

HANSCOMBE, G. E. and FORSTER, J. (1982) *Rocking the Cradle. Lesbian Mothers: A Challenge in Family Living*, London, Sheba.

HARE, J. (1994) 'Concerns and issues faced by families headed by a lesbian couple', *Families in Society*, January, pp. 27–35.

HARRIS, R. and TIMMS, N. (1993) *Secure Accommodation in Child Care*, London, Routledge.

HARRIS, R. and WEBB, D. (1987) *Welfare, Power and Juvenile Justice*, London, Tavistock.

HARTMANN, H. (1981) 'The family as the locus of gender, class and political struggle', *Signs*, **6**.

HARVEY, L. (1990) *Critical Social Research*, London, Unwin Hyman.

HASKEY, J. (1994) 'Estimated numbers of one-parent families and their prevalence in Great Britain in 1991', *Population Trends*, **78**, London, OPCS/HMSO.

HAY, C. (1995) 'Mobilization through interpellation: James Bulger, juvenile crime and the construction of a moral panic', *Social and Legal Studies*, June.

HAYDON, D. and CORTEEN, K. (1996) *Sex Education in Primary Schools: Policy and Practice*, Ormskirk, CSCSJ Research Report, Edge Hill University College.

HEARN, B. (1995) *Child and Family Support and Protection: A Practical Approach*, London, National Children's Bureau.

HEMMINGS, S. (1980) 'Horrific practices: How lesbians were presented in the newspapers of 1978', in GAY LEFT COLLECTIVE (Ed.) *Homosexuality: Power and Politics*, London, Allison and Busby.

HENDRICK, H. (1990a) *Images of Youth: Age, Class and the Male Youth Problem 1880–1920*, Oxford, Clarendon Press.

HENDRICK, H. (1990b) 'Constructions and reconstructions of British childhood: An interpretative survey, 1800 to the present', in JAMES, A. and PROUT, A. (Eds) *Constructing and Reconstructing Childhood: Contemporary Issues in the Sociological Study of Childhood*, London, Falmer Press.

HENDRICK, H. (1994) *Child Welfare in England 1872–1989*, London, Routledge.

HERMAN, E. S. and CHOMSKY, N. (1988) *Manufacturing Consent: The Political Economy of the Mass Media*, New York, Pantheon Books.

HERMAN, J. (1981) *Father-Daughter Incest*, Cambridge, Massachusetts and London, Harvard University Press.

HERNSTEIN, J. and MURRAY, C. (1994) *The Bell Curve: Intelligence and Class Structure in American Life*, New York, Free Press.

HETHERINGTON, A. (1985) *News, Newspapers and Television*, London, Macmillan.

HEWITT, P. and LEACH, P. (1993) *Social Justice, Children and Families*, London, The Commission on Social Justice/IPPR.

HEYWOOD, J. (1959) *Children in Care: The Development of the Service for the Deprived Child*, London, Routledge and Kegan Paul.

HOBSBAWN, E. (1968) *Industry and Empire*, Harmondsworth, Penguin.

HODGKIN, R. (1993) 'Measures of control in adolescent psychiatric units', *Childright*, no. 99.

HODGKIN, R. (1994) 'The right to consent to treatment', *Children UK*, Winter, pp. 4–5.

HOLLANDS, R. G. (1991) 'Working-class youth transitions: schooling and the training paradigm', in DEPARTMENT OF CULTURAL STUDIES, *Education Limited*, London, Unwin Hyman.

HOLLINGSWORTH, M. (1986) *The Press and Political Dissent*, London, Pluto Press.

HOLLY, L. (1989) *Girls and Sexuality*, Milton Keynes, Open University Press.

HOLT, J. (1973) *How Children Fail*, Harmondsworth, Penguin.

HOLT, J. (1974) *Escape from Childhood*, Harmondsworth, Penguin.

HOME OFFICE (1985) *The Cautioning of Offenders*, Circular 14, London, Home Office.

HOME OFFICE (1988) *Punishment, Custody and the Community*, London, HMSO.

HOME OFFICE (1990) *The Cautioning of Offenders*, Circular 59, London, Home Office.

HOME OFFICE (1991) *Criminal Statistics in England and Wales*, London, HMSO.

HOME OFFICE (1995) 'New arrangements for probation training and recruitment', Press Release 206/95, London, Home Office.

HOOD, R. (1992) *Race and Sentencing*, Oxford, Clarendon Press.

HOOD-WILLIAMS, J. (1990) 'Patriarchy for children: On the stability of power relations in children's lives', in CHISHOLM, L. *et al.* (Eds) *Childhood, Youth and Social Change*, London, Falmer Press.

HOUSE OF COMMONS HOME AFFAIRS COMMITTEE (1993) *Juvenile Offenders: Memoranda of Evidence*, London, HMSO.

HOWARD, M. (1993) Home Secretary's address to the Conservative Party Annual Conference, October, transcript.

HOWARD LEAGUE (1995a) *Secure Training Centres Repeating Past Failures*, London, The Howard League for Penal Reform.

HOWARD LEAGUE (1995b) *Banged Up, Beaten Up, Cutting Up: Report of the Howard League Commission of Inquiry into Violence in Penal Institutions for Teenagers under 18*, London, The Howard League for Penal Reform.

HOWARD LEAGUE (1995c) *Child Offenders: UK and International Practice*, London, The Howard League for Penal Reform.

HUDSON, A. (1983) 'The welfare state and adolescent femininity', *Youth and Policy*, **2** (1), Summer.

HUDSON, A. (1988) 'Boys will be boys: Masculinism and the juvenile justice system', *Critical Social Policy*, **21**, pp. 31–48.

HUDSON, B. (1984) 'Femininity and adolescence', in McROBBIE, A. and NAVA, M. (Eds) *Gender and Education*, Basingstoke, Macmillan.

HUDSON, F. and INEICHEN, B. (1991) *Taking It Lying Down: Sexuality and Teenage Motherhood*, London, Macmillan.

HUNT, E. H. (1981) *British Labour History, 1815–1914*, London, Weidenfeld and Nicolson.

HUTTON, W. (1995) *The State We're In: Why Britain Is in Crisis and How to Overcome It*, London, Jonathan Cape.

IGNATIEFF, M. (1978) *A Just Measure of Pain: The Penitentiary in the Industrial Revolution, 1750–1850*, London, Macmillan.

ILLICH, I. (1971) *Deschooling Society*, Harmondsworth, Penguin.

IVORY, M. (1991) 'Compulsory or by consent?', *Community Care*, no. 874, 1 August, p. 8.

JACKSON, S. (1982) *Childhood and Sexuality*, London, Basil Blackwell.

JAFFA, T. and DESZERY, A. M. (1989) 'Reasons for admission to an adolescent unit', *Journal of Adolescence*, **12**, pp. 187–95.

JAMES, A. and PROUT, A. (1990) *Constructing and Reconstructing Childhood: Contemporary Issues in the Sociological Study of Childhood*, London, Falmer Press.

JAMESON, N. and ALLISON, E. (1995) *Strangeways 1990: A Serious Disturbance*, London, Larkin Publications.

JEFFREY-POULTER, S. (1991) *Peers, Queers and Commons: The Struggle for Gay Law Reform from 1950 to the Present*, London, Routledge.

JENKINS, M. (1980) *The General Strike of 1842*, London, Lawrence and Wishart.

JOLLY, S. and SANDLAND, R. (1994) 'Political correctness and the adoption white paper', *Family Law*, January, pp. 30–32.

JONES, C. (1983) *State Social Work and the Working Class*, London, Macmillan.

JONES, C. and MAHONY, P. (Eds) (1989) *Learning Our Lines: Sexuality and Social Control in Education*, London, The Women's Press.

JONES, C. L., TEPPERMAN, L. and WILSON, S. J. (1995) *The Futures of the Family*, Englewood Cliffs, New Jersey, Prentice Hall.

JONES, G. and WALLACE, C. (1990) 'Beyond individualisation: What sort of social change?', in CHISHOLM, L. *et al.* (Eds) *Childhood, Youth and Social Change: A Comparative Perspective*, London, Falmer Press.

JONES, P. (1985) 'Remand decisions at magistrates courts', in MAXON, D. (Ed.) *Managing Criminal Justice: A Collection of Papers*, London, HMSO.

JORDANOVA, L. (1989) 'Children in history: Concepts of nature and society', in SCARRE, G. (Ed.) *Children, Parents and Politics*, Cambridge, Cambridge University Press.

JOSEPH ROWNTREE FOUNDATION (1995) *Income and Wealth*, York, Joseph Rowntree Foundation.

JOSEPH ROWNTREE FOUNDATION (1995) *Inquiry Into Income and Welfare*, York, Joseph Rowntree Foundation.

References

KEEGAN. EAMON M. (1994) 'Institutionalizing children and adolescents in private psychiatric hospitals', *Social Work*, **39** (5), September, pp. 588–94.

KELLY, L. (1988) *Surviving Sexual Violence*, Cambridge, Polity Press.

KENNEDY, H. (1995) 'Preface to the report of the Howard League Commission of inquiry into violence in penal institutions for young people', *Banged Up, Beaten Up, Cutting Up*, London, Howard League for Penal Reform.

KERR, M. (1958) *The People of Ship Street*, London, Routledge and Kegan Paul.

KIERNAN, K. and ESTAUGH, V. (1993) *Cohabitation: Extra-marital Childbearing and Social Policy*, Occasional Paper 17, London, Family Policy Studies Centre.

KING, D. S. (1987) *The New Right: Politics, Markets and Citizenship*, London, Macmillan.

KITZINGER, C. and WILKINSON, S. (1993) 'Theorizing heterosexuality', in WILKINSON, S. and KITZINGER, C. (Eds) *Heterosexuality: A Feminism and Psychology Reader*, London, Sage.

KITZINGER, J. (1988) 'Defending innocence: Ideologies of childhood', *Feminist Review*, **28**, Spring, pp. 77–87.

KITZINGER, J. (1990) 'Who are you kidding? Children and sociology in the UK', in CHISHOLM, L. *et al.* (Eds) *Childhood, Youth and Social Change*, London, Falmer Press.

KOVARIK, J. (1994) 'The space and time of children at the interface of psychology and sociology', in QVORTRUP, J. *et al.* (Eds) *Childhood Matters: Social Theory, Practice and Politics*, Aldershot, Avebury.

KRÜGER, H. (1990) 'Caught between homogenization and disintegration: Changes in the life-phase "youth" in West Germany since 1945', in CHISHOLM, L. *et al.* (Eds) *Childhood, Youth and Social Change: A Comparative Perspective*, London, Falmer Press.

KUPER, J. and WILLIAMSON, J. (1993) *Treated with Humanity and Respect? Conditions for Young People in Custody*, London, Children's Legal Centre.

KURTZ, Z. (1992) *With Health in Mind: Mental Health Care for Children and Young People*, Action for Sick Children in Association with South West Thames Regional Health Authority.

KURTZ, Z., THORNES, R. and WOLKIND, S. (1994) *Services for the Mental Health of Children and Young People in England: A National Review*, London: Maudsley Hospital and South Thames (West) Regional Health Authority.

LAND, H. (1976) 'Women: Supporters or supported?', in BARKER, D. L. and ALLEN, S. (Eds) *Sexual Divisions and Society: Process and Change*, London, Tavistock.

LAND, H. (1978) 'Who cares for the family?', *Journal of Social Policy*, **7** (3), pp. 257–84.

LAND, H. (1983) 'Poverty and gender', in BROWN, M. (Ed.) *The Structure of Disadvantage*, London, Heinemann.

LAND, H. and ROSE, H. (1985) 'Compulsory altruism for some or an altruistic society for all', in BEAN, P. (Ed.) *In Defence of Welfare*, London, Tavistock.

LANDAU, S. *et al.* (1983) 'Selecting delinquents for cautioning in the London Metropolitan Area', *British Journal of Criminology*, **23**.

LASLETT, P. (1977) *Family Life and Illicit Love in Earlier Generations*, Cambridge, Cambridge University Press.

LASLETT, P. and WALL, R. (Eds) (1972) *Household and Family in Past Time*, Cambridge, Cambridge University Press.

LAWSON, E. (1991) 'Are Gillick rights under threat?', *Childright*, no. 80, pp. 17–21.

LAWTON, D. (1977) *Education and Social Justice*, London, Sage.

LAWTON, D. (1994) *The Tory Mind on Education, 1979–1994*, London, Falmer Press.

LEES, S. (1986) *Losing Out: Sexuality and Adolescent Girls*, London, Hutchinson.

LEES, S. (1993) *Sugar and Spice: Sexuality and Adolescent Girls*, Harmondsworth, Penguin.

LEONARD, D. (1990) 'Persons in their own right: Children and sociology in the UK', in CHISHOLM, L. *et al.* (Eds) *Childhood, Youth and Social Change*, London, Falmer Press.

LEVY, E. F. (1992) 'Strengthening the coping resources of lesbian families', *Families in Society*, January, pp. 23–31.

LEWIS, J. (1983) *Women's Welfare/Women's Rights*, London, Croom Helm.

LEWIS, J. (1986) 'Anxieties about the family and the relationships between parents, children and the state in twentieth century England', in RICHARD, M. and LIGHT, P. (Eds) *Children of Social Worlds*, Cambridge, Polity Press.

LIEBLING, A. (1992) *Suicides in Prison*, London, Routledge.

LIEBLING, A. and KRARUP, A. (1993) *Suicide Attempts and Self Injury in Male Prisons*, London, Report submitted to the Home Office.

LONEY, M. (1989) 'Child abuse in a social context', in STAINTON-ROGERS, W., HARVEY, D. and ASH, E., *Child Abuse and Neglect: Facing the Challenge*, London, B.T. Batsford (in association with Open University Press).

MAC AN GHAILL, M. (1994) *The Making of Men: Masculinities, Sexualities and Schooling*, Buckingham, Open University Press.

MACLEOD, M. and SARAGA, E. (1988) 'Challenging the orthodoxy: Towards a feminist theory and practice', *Feminist Review*, no. 28, January.

MACLURE, J. S. (1969) *Educational Documents: England and Wales 1816–1968*, 2nd Edn, London, Methuen.

MACLURE, S. (Ed.) (1992) *Education Re-formed: A Guide to the Education Reform Act*, 3rd Edn, London, Hodder & Stoughton.

MACNICOL, J. (1980) *The Movement for Family Allowances 1918–45: A Study in Social Policy Development*, London, Heinemann.

McEwan, D. (1991) 'Hustled by history: choices before teachers in a progressive school', in Department of Cultural Studies, *Education Limited*, London, Unwin Hyman.

McIntosh, M. (1981) 'Sexual division of labour and the subordination of women', in Young, K. *et al.* (eds) *Of Marriage and the Market: Women's Subordination in International Perspective*, London, CSE Books.

McLaren, P. (1986) *Schooling as a Ritual Performance*, London, Routledge and Kegan Paul.

McNay, I. and Ozga, J. (1985) *Policy Making in Education: The Breakdown of Consensus*, Oxford, Pergamon Press.

Makrinioti, D. (1994) 'Conceptualisation of childhood in a welfare state: A critical reappraisal', in Qvortrup, J. *et al.* (Eds) *Childhood Matters: Social Theory, Practice and Politics*, Aldershot, Avebury.

Malek, M. (1991) *Psychiatric Admissions: A Report on Young People Entering Residential Psychiatric Care*, London, The Children's Society.

Malinowski, B. (1927) *Sex and Repression in Savage Society*, London, Routledge and Kegan Paul.

Mama, A. (1989) *The Hidden Struggle: Statutory and Voluntary Sector Responses to Violence Against Black Women in the Home*, London, London Race and Housing Research Unit.

Manton, J. (1976) *Mary Carpenter and the Children of the Streets*, London, Heinemann.

Margolin, C. R. (1978) 'Salvation versus liberation: The movement for children's rights in an historical context', *Social Problems*, **25** (4).

Marsh, D. (1980) *The Welfare State*, London, Longman.

Marshall, T. H. (1965) *Social Policy*, London, Hutchinson.

Masson, J. (1984) *The Assault on Truth: Freud's Suppression of the Seduction Theory*, New York, Farrar, Straus & Giroux.

Masson, J. (1991) 'Adolescent crisis and parental power', *Family Law*, December, pp. 528–31.

Masson, J. (1992) *Against Therapy*, London, Fontana.

Measor, L. (1989) '"Are you coming to see some dirty films today?" Sex education and adolescent sexuality', in Holly, L. (Ed.) *Girls and Sexuality*, Milton Keynes, Open University Press.

Middleton, S., Ashworth, K. and Walker, R. (1994) *Family Fortunes: Pressures on Parents and Children in the 1990s*, London, Child Poverty Action Group.

Miller, A. (1983) *For Your Own Good: Hidden Cruelty in Childrearing and the Roots of Violence*, London, Faber and Faber.

Miller, A. (1985) *Thou Shalt Not Be Aware*, London, Pluto Press.

Miller, A. (1990) *Banished Knowledge: Facing Childhood Injuries*, London, Virago.

Millett, K. (1970) *Sexual Politics*, London, Virago.

Mishra, R. (1984) *The Welfare State in Crisis*, Brighton, Wheatsheaf.

MOREL, M. (1989) 'Reflections on some recent french literature on the history of childhood', in *Continuity and Change: A Journal of Social Structure, Law and Demography in Past Societies*, **4** (2), pp. 323–37.

MORGAN, P. (1986) 'Feminist attempts to sack father: A case of unfair dismissal?', in ANDERSON, D. and DAWSON, G. (Eds) *Family Portraits*, London, Social Affairs Unit.

MORGAN, P. (1995) *Farewell to the Family? Public Policy and Family Breakdown in Britain and the USA*, London, Insitute of Economic Affairs.

MORRIS, A. and MCISAAC, A. (1978) *Juvenile Justice? The Practice of Social Welfare*, London, Heinemann.

MORRIS, A. and GILLER, H. (Eds) (1983) *Providing Criminal Justice for Children*, London, Edward Arnold.

MORT, F. (1980) 'Sexuality: Regulation and contestation', in Gay Left Collective (Eds) *Homosexuality: Power and Politics*, London, Allison and Busby.

MORRISH, I. (1972) *The Sociology of Education: An Introduction*, London, Allen & Unwin.

MORT, F. (1987) *Dangerous Sexualities*, London, Routledge.

MOUNT, F. (1982) *The Subversive Family*, London, Jonathan Cape.

MOUNTAIN, A. (1988) *Womanpower: A Handbook for Women Working with Young Women in Trouble*, Leicester, National Youth Bureau.

MUNCIE, J. (1981) *Law and Disorder: Histories of Crime and Justice*, D335 Block 2, Part 4, Youth and the Reforming Zeal, Milton Keynes, Open University Press.

MUNCIE, J. (1984) *The Trouble with Kids Today: Postwar Youth and Crime in Postwar Britain*, London, Hutchinson & Co.

MURDOCK, G. (1949) *Social Structure*, New York, Macmillan.

MURRAY, C. (1984) *Losing Ground: American Social Policy 1950–80*, New York, Basic Books.

MURRAY, C. (1989) *In Pursuit of Happiness and Good Government*, New York, Basic Books.

MURRAY, C. (1990) *The Emerging British Underclass*, London, Institute of Economic Affairs.

MURRAY, C. (1993) 'Keep it in the family', *Sunday Times*, 14 November.

MURRAY, C. (1994) *Underclass: The Crisis Deepens*, London, Institute of Economic Affairs.

MUSGROVE, P. W. (1965) *The Sociology of Education*, London, Methuen.

NACRO (1992) *Young Black People in Custody: A Review of Home Office Prison Statistics*, London, NACRO.

NACRO (1995) *Crisis in Custody: A Survey of Juveniles Remanded to Custody While Awaiting Trial*, London, NACRO Youth Crime Section.

NAPCE (1993) 'Responses to department for education revision of Circular 11/87: Sex education in schools, National Association for Pastoral Care in Education, Coventry, University of Warwick.

References

NATIONAL CURRICULUM COUNCIL (1990) *The Whole Curriculum*, York, National Curriculum Council.

NATIONAL INTERMEDIATE TREATMENT FEDERATION (NITFED) (1986) *Anti-Racist Practice for Intermediate Treatment*, London, NITFED.

NAVA, M. (1988) 'Cleveland and the press: Outrage and anxiety in the reporting of child sexual abuse', *Feminist Review*, no. 28, January.

NCB (1994) *Sex Education Forum Fact Sheet 3*, London, National Children's Bureau.

NCCL (1991) *A People's Charter: Liberty's Bill of Rights*, London, Liberty.

NCH ACTION FOR CHILDREN (1995) *Factfile '95*, London, NCH Action for Children.

NELSON, S. (1982) *Incest: Fact and Myth*, Edinburgh, Stramullion.

NEWBURN, T. (1995) *Crime and Criminal Justice Policy*, London, Methuen.

NEWELL, P. (1989) *Children Are People Too*, London, Bedford Square Press.

NEWELL, P. (1989) 'Spare the Rod . . . ?' *Childright*, no. 60.

NHS HEALTH ADVISORY SERVICE (1986) *Bridges Over Troubled Waters: A Report on Services for Disturbed Adolescents*, London, HMSO.

NHS HEALTH ADVISORY SERVICE (1995) *Together We Stand: The Commissioning, Role and Management of Child and Adolescent Mental Health Services*, London, HMSO.

NIESTROJ, B. (1989) 'Some recent German literature on socialisation and childhood in past times', *Continuity and Change: A Journal of Social Structure, Law and Demography in Past Societies*, **4** (2), pp. 339–57.

OAKLEY, A. (1979) *From here to Maternity: Becoming a Mother*, Harmondsworth, Penguin.

O'BRIEN, M. (1981) *The Politics of Reproduction*, London, Routledge and Kegan Paul.

O'DONOVAN, K. (1985) *Sexual Divisions in Law*, London, Weidenfeld & Nicolson.

OFFICE FOR STANDARDS IN EDUCATION (1993) *Education for Disaffected Pupils*, London, OFSTED.

OGDEN, J. (1991) 'Care or control?', *Social Work Today*, 4 July, p. 9.

O'HARA, M. (1991) 'The rights and wrongs of children: Child sexual abuse and the reassertion of fathers' rights', *Trouble and Strife*, no. 20, Spring, pp. 28–34.

OPCS (1990) *Marriage and Divorce Statistics 1837–1983*, London, HMSO.

OPCS (1994a) *1992 Marriage and Divorce Statistics: England and Wales*, London, HMSO.

OPCS (1994b) *1992 General Household Survey*, London, HMSO.

OPPENHEIM, C. (1993) *Poverty: The Facts* (2nd Edn) London, Child Poverty Action Group.

ORWELL, G. (1954) *Nineteen Eighty-Four*, Harmondsworth, Penguin.

PAHL, J. (Ed.) (1985) *Private Violence and Public Policy*, London, Routledge and Kegan Paul.

PAQUETTE, J. (1991) *Social Purpose and Schooling: Alternatives, Agendas and Issues*, London, Falmer Press.

PARKER, R. (1988) 'Children', in SINCLAIR, I. (Ed.) *Residential Care: The Research Reviewed*, London, HMSO.

PARSONS, T. (1949) 'The social structure of the family', in ANSHEN, R. (Ed.) *The Family: Its Function and Destiny*, New York, Harper.

PARSONS, T. (1955) 'The American family', in PARSONS, T. and BALES, R., *Family, Socialization and Interaction Process*, Glencoe, IL, Free Press.

PARTON N. (1985) *The Politics of Child Abuse*, London, Macmillan.

PARTON, N. (1991) *Governing the Family: Child Care, Child Protection and the State*, London, Macmillan.

PEARSON, G. (1975) *The Deviant Imagination*, London, Macmillan.

PEARSON, G. (1983) *Hooligan: A History of Respectable Fears*, London, Macmillan.

PEARSON, G. (1993/1994) 'Youth crime and moral decline: Permissiveness and tradition', *The Magistrate*, December/January.

PENAL AFFAIRS CONSORTIUM (1994) *The Case Against the Secure Training Order*, London, Penal Affairs Consortium.

PENAL AFFAIRS CONSORTIUM (1995) *Boot Camps for Young Offenders*, London, Penal Affairs Consortium.

PENAL AFFAIRS CONSORTIUM (1996) *Young Offenders and the Glasshouse*, London, Penal Affairs Consortium.

PHILLIPS, A. (1993) *The Trouble with Boys: Parenting the Men of the Future*, London, Pandora.

PIKE, E. (1996) *Human Documents of the Industrial Revolution in Britain*, London, Allen and Unwin.

PINCHBECK, I. and HEWITT, M. (1969) and (1973) *Children in English Society 1780–1880* (2 Vols), London, Routledge and Kegan Paul.

PITTS, J. (1988) *The Politics of Juvenile Crime*, London, Sage Publications.

PITTS, J. (1990) *Working with Young Offenders*, London, Macmillan.

POLLOCK, L. (1983) *Forgotten Children*, Cambridge, Cambridge University Press.

POSTMAN, N. (1982) *The Disappearance of Childhood*, New York, Delacourt Press.

PRATT, J. (1985) 'Juvenile justice, social work and social control: The need for positive thinking', *British Journal of Social Work*, **15**.

PRATT, J. (1987) 'A revisionist history of intermediate treatment', *British Journal of Social Work*, **17**.

PROUT, A. and JAMES, A. (Eds) (1990) *Constructing and Reconstructing Childhood*, London, Falmer Press.

QUEST, C. (Ed.) (1992) *Equal Opportunities: A Feminist Fallacy*, London, Institute of Economic Affairs.

QUEST, C. (Ed.) (1994) *Liberating Women from Modern Feminism*, London, Institute of Economic Affairs.

QVORTRUP, J. (1994) 'Childhood matters: An introduction', in QVORTRUP, J. *et al.* (Eds) *Childhood Matters: Social Theory, Practice and Politics*, Aldershot, Avebury.

RADFORD, J. (1995–96) 'Twin leaks and hackney outings: The Kingsmead School affair', *Trouble and Strife*, Winter, pp. 3–8.

RADFORD, J. and RUSSELL, D. E. H. (Eds) (1992) *Femicide: The Politics of Woman Killing*, Buckingham, Open University Press.

REDMAN, P. (1994) 'Shifting ground: Rethinking sexuality education', in EPSTEIN, D. (Ed.) *Challenging Lesbian and Gay Inequalities in Education*, Buckingham, Open University Press.

REID, I. (1978) *Sociological Perspectives on School and Education*, London, Open Books.

REINHARZ, S. (1993) 'The principles of feminist research: A matter of Debate', in KRAMARAE, C. and SPENDER, D. (Eds) *The Knowledge Explosion: Generations of Feminist Scholarship*, London, Harvester Wheatsheaf.

RICH, A. (1977) *Of Woman Born: Motherhood as Experience and Institution*, London, Virago.

RILEY, D. (1983) *War in the Nursery: Theories of the Child and Mother*, London, Virago.

ROCK, P. (1973) 'New eternal recurrence', in COHEN, S. and YOUNG, J., *The Manufacture of News: Social Problems, Deviance and the Mass Media*, London, Constable/Sage.

RODGER, J. (1995) 'Family policy or moral regulation?', *Critical Social Policy*, Issue 43, **15** (1), Summer, pp. 5–25.

RODHAM, H. (1976) 'Children under the law', in SKOLNICK, A. (Ed.) *Rethinking Childhood*, Boston, MA, Little Brown and Co.

ROONEY, B. (1987) *Racism and Resistance to Change: A Study of the Black Social Workers Project in Liverpool Social Services Department*, Liverpool, Merseyside Area Profile Group.

ROSE, L. (1991) *The Erosion of Childhood: Child Oppression in Britain 1860–1918*, London, Routledge.

ROSE, N. (1979) 'The psychological complex: mental measurement and social administration', *Ideology and Consciousness*, no. 5, Spring, pp. 5–68.

ROSE, N. (1985) *The Psychological Complex: Psychology, Politics and Society in England 1869–1939*, London, Routledge and Kegan Paul.

ROSE, N. (1987) 'Beyond the public/private division: Law, power and the family', *Journal of Law and Society*, **14** (1), Spring.

ROSE N. (1989) 'Individualizing psychology', in SHOTTER, J. and GERGEN, K. J. (Eds) *Texts of Identity*, London, Sage.

ROSE, N. (1990) *Governing the Soul: The Shaping of the Private Self*, London, Routledge.

ROTHMAN, D. J. (1978) 'Introduction' and 'The state as parent', in GAYLIN, W. *et al.* (Eds) *Doing Good: The Limits of Benevolence*, New York, Pantheon.

ROTHMAN, D. J. (1980) *Conscience and Convenience: The Asylum and Its Alternatives in Progressive America*, Boston, MA, Little Brown.

ROUSSEAU, J. J. (1756) *Emile*, tr. FOXELY, B., London, Everyman's Library.

RUDDOCK, M. (1991) 'A receptacle for public anger', in FRANKLIN, B. and PARTON, N. (Eds) *Social Work, the Media and Public Relations*, London, Routledge and Kegan Paul.

RUSCHE, G. and KIRCHHEIMER, O. (1938) *Punishment and the Social Structure*, New York, Russell and Russell.

RUSH, F. (1980) *The Best Kept Secret: Sexual Abuse of Children*, New York, McGraw-Hill.

RUSSELL, D. (1995) *Women, Madness and Medicine*, Cambridge, Polity Press.

RUTHERFORD, A. (1986) *Growing Out of Crime: Society and Young People in Trouble*, Harmondsworth, Penguin.

RUTHERFORD, A. (1992) *Growing Out of Crime: The New Era*, Winchester, Waterside Press.

RUTHERFORD, A. (1995) 'Signposting the future of juvenile justice policy in England and Wales', in Howard League for Penal Reform, *Child Offenders UK and International Practice*, London, Howard League.

RUTTER, M. (1977) *Helping Troubled Children*, Harmondsworth, Penguin.

SANDERS, S. and SPRAGGS, G. (1989) 'Section 28 and education', in JONES, C. and MAHONY, P. (Eds) *Learning Our Lines: Sexuality and Social Control in Education*, London, The Women's Press.

SAPSFORD, R. (1993) 'Understanding people: The growth of an expertise', in CLARKE, J. (Ed.) *A Crisis in Care? Challenges to Social Work*, London, Sage/Open University.

SCARRE, G. (Ed.) (1989) *Children, Parents and Politics*, Cambridge, Cambridge University Press.

SCHOOLS COUNCIL (1982) *Multicultural Education*, London, Schools Council.

SCRATON, P. (1982) 'Policing and institutionalised racism on Merseyside', in COWELL, D. *et al.* (Eds) *Policing the Riots*, London, Junction Books.

SCRATON, P. (1985) *The State of the Police*, London, Pluto.

SCRATON, P. (Ed.) (1987) *Law, Order and the Authoritarian State*, Milton Keynes, Open University Press.

SCRATON, P. (1989) *Unreasonable Force: Class Marginality and the Political Autonomy of the Police*, University of Lancaster, PhD Thesis.

SCRATON, P. (1990) 'Scientific knowledge or masculine discourse? Challenging patriarchy in criminology', in GELSHORPE, L. and MORRIS, A. (Eds) *Feminist Perspectives in Criminology*, Buckingham, Open University Press.

SCRATON, P. and CHADWICK, K. (1991) 'The theoretical and political priorities of critical criminology', in STENSON, K. and COWELL, D. (Eds) *The Politics of Crime Control*, London, Sage.

SCRATON, P., JEMPHREY, A. and COLEMAN, S. (1995) *No Last Rights: The Denial of Justice and the Promotion of Myth in the Aftermath of the Hillsborough Disaster*, Liverpool, Alden Press/LCC.

References

SCRATON, P., SIM, J. and SKIDMORE, P. (1991) *Prisons Under Protest*, Buckingham, Open University Press.

SCRUTON, R. (1986) *Sexual Desire*, London, Weidenfeld & Nicolson.

SEARS, J. T. (1992) 'The impact of culture and ideology on the construction of gender and sexual identities', in SEARS, J. T. (Ed.) *Sexuality and the Curriculum: The Politics and Practices of Sexuality Education*, New York, NY Teachers College, Columbia University.

SEARS, J. T. (1992) 'Dilemmas and possibilities of sexuality education: Reproducing the body politic', in SEARS, J. T. (Ed.) *Sexuality and the Curriculum: The Politics and Practices of Sexuality Education*, New York, NY Teachers College, Columbia University.

SEGAL, L. (1990) *Slow Motion: Changing Masculinities, Changing Men*, London, Virago.

SEGALMAN, R. and MARSLAND, D. (1989) *Cradle to Grave*, London, Macmillan/Social Affairs Unit.

SELECT COMMISSION ON RACE RELATIONS AND IMMIGRATION (1973; 1977) *Education: Vol. 1, Report*, London, HMSO.

SEX EDUCATION FORUM (1992) *An Inquiry into Sex Education*, London, National Children's Bureau.

SGRITTA, G. (1994) 'The generalisation divisions of welfare: Equity and conflict', in QVORTRUP, J. *et al.* (Eds) *Childhood Matters: Social Theory, Practice and Politics*, Aldershot, Avebury.

SHAMGAR-HANDELMAN, L. (1994) 'To whom does childhood belong', in QVORTRUP, J. *et al.* (Eds) *Childhood Matters: Social Theory, Practice and Politics*, Aldershot, Avebury.

SHOTTON, J. (1993) *No Master High or Low: Libertarian Education and Schooling 1890–1990*, London, Libertarian Education.

SHOWSTACK-SASSOON, A. (Ed.) (1987) *Women and the State*, London, Hutchinson.

SINDALL, R. (1990) *Street Violence in the Nineteenth Century*, Leicester, Leicester University Press.

SINGER, E. (1992) *Child-care and the Psychology of Development*, London, Routledge.

SMART, C. and SMART, B. (1978) *Women, Sexuality and Social Control*, London, Routledge and Kegan Paul.

SMART, C. (1984) *The Ties That Bind*, London, Routledge and Kegan Paul.

SMART, C. (1989) 'Power and the politics of child custody', in SMART, C. and SEVENHUIJSEN, S. (Eds) *Child Custody and the Politics of Gender*, London, Routledge.

SMART, C. (1991) 'Securing the family? Rhetoric and policy in the field of social security', in LONEY, M. *et al.* (Eds) *The State of the Market: Politics and Welfare in Contemporary Britain*, London, Sage/Open University.

SMITH, A. M. (1995) 'A symptomology of an authoritarian discourse', in CARTER, E. *et al.* (Eds) *Cultural Remix*, London, Lawrence and Wishart.

SMITH, D. E. (1973) 'Women's perspective as a radical critique of sociology', *Sociological Inquiry*, **44** (1).

SMITH, T. and NOBLE, M. (1995) *Education Divides: Poverty and Schooling in the 1990s*, London, Child Poverty Action Group.

SONE, K. (1994) 'The forgotten children', *Community Care*, no. 1014, 30 April, pp. 22–3.

STAINTON ROGERS, R. and STAINTON ROGERS, W. (1992) *Stories of Childhood*, London, Harvester Wheatsheaf.

STANKO, E. A. (1985) *Intimate Intrusions: Women's Experiences of Violence*, London, Routledge and Kegan Paul.

STANLEY, L. and WISE, S. (1993) *Breaking Out: Feminist Consciousness and Feminist Research*, London, Routledge and Kegan Paul.

STEDMAN JONES, G. (1977) *Outcast London*, Oxford, Oxford University Press.

STEINBERG, D. (1981) 'Two years referrals to a regional adolescent unit: Some implications for psychiatric services', *Social Science and Medicine*, **15**.

STEVENSON, J. and COOK, C. (1994) *Britain in the Depression: Society and Politics 1929–39*, London, Longman.

STEVENSON, K. (1994) 'The provision of sex education in schools: The new DFE guidelines', in *Childright*, no. 109, September.

STEWART, G. and STEWART, J. (1993) *Social Circumstances of Young Offenders Under Supervision*, London, Association of Chief Officers of Probation.

STOLTENBERG, J. (1991) *Refusing to Be a Man*, London, Fontana.

STONE, L. (1974) *The Massacre of the Innocents*, New York, New York Review of Books.

SURANSKY, V. (1982) *The Erosion of Childhood*, Chicago, IL, University of Chicago Press.

SWANN LORD, M. (1985) *Education for All: The Report of the Committee of Inquiry into the Education of Children from Ethnic Minority Groups*, Cmnd 9453, London, (Cmnd 9453) HMSO.

TAPPER, T. and SALTER, B. (1978) *Education and the Political Order: Changing Patterns of Class Control*, London, Macmillan.

TAYLOR, S. J. (1992) *Shock! Horror! The Tabloids in Action*, London, Black Swan.

THANE, P. (1981) 'Childhood in history', in KING, M. (Ed.) *Childhood Welfare and Justice*, London, Batsford.

THOMAS, P. and COSTIGAN, R. (1990) *Promoting Homosexuality: Section 28 of the Local Government Act*, Cardiff, Cardiff Law School.

THOMPSON, E. P. (1968) *The Making of the English Working Class*, Harmondsworth, Penguin.

THOMSON, R. (1993) 'Unholy alliances: The recent politics of sex education', in BRISTOW, J. and WILSON, A. (Eds) *Activating Theory*, London, Lawrence and Wishart.

THORNE, B. (1982) 'Feminist rethinking of the family: An overview', in THORNE, B. and YALLOM, M. (Eds) *Rethinking the Family: Some Feminist Questions*, Harlow, Longman.

THORNTON, D. (1984) *Tougher Regimes in Detention Centres: Report of an Evaluation by the Young Offender Psychology Unit*, London, Home Office.

THORPE, D., SMITH, D., GREEN, C. and PALEY, J. (1980) *Out of Care*, London, Allen & Unwin.

TOBIAS, J. (1967) *Crime and Industrial Society in the Nineteenth Century*, London, Batsford.

TORKINGTON, P. (1983) *The Racial Politics of Health: A Liverpool Profile*, Liverpool, Merseyside Area Profile Group.

TORKINGTON, P. (1991) *Black Health a Political Issue*, Liverpool, Catholic Association for Racial Justice and Liverpool Institute of Higher Education.

TROYNA, B. (1993) *Racism and Education*, London, Routledge.

TUMIM, S. (1990) *Report of a Review by Her Majesty's Inspector of Prisons for England and Wales of Suicide and Self-Harm in Prison Service Establishments in England and Wales*, London, HMSO.

TUMIM, S. (1992) *HM Chief Inspector of Prisons, Annual Report 1990–91*, London, HMSO.

TUNSTALL, J. (1971) *Journalists at Work*, London, Constable.

UNGERSON, C. (Ed.) (1990) *Gender and Caring*, London, Harvester Wheatsheaf.

UNITED NATIONS (1985) *The Beijing Rules: The United Nations Standard Minimum Rules for the Administration of Juvenile Justice*, New York, United Nations.

UNITED NATIONS (1989) *The United Nations Convention on the Rights of the Child*, New York, United Nations.

UNITED NATIONS (1990) *The Riyadh Guidelines: The United Nations Guidelines for the Prevention of Juvenile Delinquency*, New York, United Nations.

UNITED NATIONS COMMITTEE ON THE RIGHTS OF THE CHILD (1995) *Eighth Session. Consideration of Reports Submitted by States Parties Under Article 44 of the Convention*, New York, United Nations.

URWIN, C. and SHARLAND, E. (1992) 'From bodies to minds in childcare literature: Advice to parents in inter-war britain', in COOTER, R. (Ed.) *In the Name of the Child: Health and Welfare 1880–1940*, London, Routledge.

UTTING, D. (1995) *Family and Parenthood: Supporting families, preventing breakdown*, York, Joseph Rowntree Foundation.

VAN EVERY, J. (1991) 'Who is "the family"? The assumptions of British social policy', *Critical Social Policy*, **11** (3), pp. 62–75.

VIOLENCE AGAINST CHILDREN STUDY GROUP (1990) *Taking Child Abuse Seriously*, London, Unwin Hyman.

WADE, E. (1985) 'The miners and the media: Themes of newspaper reporting', in SCRATON, P. and THOMAS, P. (Eds) *The State v. The People: Lessons from the Coal Dispute*, Oxford, JLS/Basil Blackwell.

WALBY, S. (1990) *Theorizing Patriarchy*, Oxford, Blackwell.

WALKER, S. and BARTON, L. (Eds) (1983) *Gender, Class and Education*, London, Falmer Press.

WALKERDINE, V. (1984) 'Developmental psychology and the child-centred pedagogy', in HENRIQUES, J., HOLLOWAY, W., URWIN, C., VENN, C. and WALKERDINE, V., *Changing the Subject: Psychology, Social Regulation and Subjectivity*, London, Methuen.

WARDLE, D. (1974) *The Rise of the Schooled Society: The History of Schooling in England*, London, Routledge and Kegan Paul.

WATNEY, S. (1991) 'Schools out', in FUSS, D. (Ed.) *Inside/Out*, London, Routledge.

WEEKS, J. (1989) *Sex, Politics and Society: The Regulation of Sexuality Since 1800*, London, Longman.

WEEKS, J. (1993) 'An unfinished revolution: Sexuality in the Twentieth Century', in HARWOOD, V. (Ed.) *Pleasure Principles*, London, Lawrence and Wishart.

WHATLEY, M. H. (1992) 'Whose sexuality is it anyway?', in SEARS, J. T. (Ed.) *Sexuality and the Curriculum: The Politics and Practices of Sexuality Education*, New York, NY Teachers College, Columbia University.

WICKS, M. (1991) 'Family matters and public policy', in LONEY, M. *et al.* (Eds) *The State or the Market: Politics and Welfare in Contemporary Britain*, London, Sage/Open University.

WILLIAMS, J. (1993) 'What Is a profession? Experience versus expertise', in WALMSLEY, J. *et al.* (Eds) *Health, Welfare and Practice: Reflecting on Roles and Relationships*, London, Sage/Open University.

WILLIAMSON, H. (1993) 'Youth policy in the United Kingdom and the marginalisation of young people', *Youth and Policy*, **40**, pp. 33–48.

WILLIS, C. F. (1983) *The Use, Effectiveness and Impact of Police Stop and Search Powers*, London, Home Office Research Unit HMSO.

WILLIS, P. E. (1977) *Learning to Labour: How Working Class Kids Get Working Class Jobs*, London, Gower.

WILLMOTT, P. and YOUNG, M. (1971) *Family and Class in a London Suburb*, London, New English Library.

WILLMOTT, P. and YOUNG, M. (1986) *Family and Kinship in East London*, London, Routledge.

WILSON, E. (1977) *Women and the Welfare State*, London, Tavistock.

WILTON, T. (1995) *Lesbian Studies: Setting an Agenda*, London, Routledge.

WINN, M. (1983) *Children Without Childhood*, New York, Pantheon Books.

WINNICOTT, D. (1957) *The Child and the Family; and the Child and the Outside World*, London, Tavistock.

WINTERSBERGER, H. (1994) 'Costs and benefits – The economics of childhood', in QVORTRUP, J. *et al.* (Eds) *Childhood Matters, Social Theory, Practice and Politics*, Aldershot, Avebury.

WOOLF REPORT (1991) *Prison Disturbance, April 1990: Report of an Inquiry*, London, HMSO.

WOLPE, A-M. (1988) *Within School Walls: The Role of Discipline, Sexuality and the Curriculum*, London, Routledge.

WOOD, J. (1984) 'Groping towards sexism: Boys' sex talk', in MCROBBIE, A. and NAVA, M. (Eds) *Gender and Generation*, Basingstoke, Macmillan.

WOODS, P. (1979) *The Divided School*, London, Routledge and Kegan Paul.

WOODS, P. (Ed.) (1980a) *Teacher Strategies*, London, Croom Helm.

WOODS, P. (Ed.) (1980b) *Pupil Strategies*, London, Croom Helm.

WOODS, P. (1990) *The Happiest Days? How Pupils Cope with Schools*, London, Falmer Press.

WRIGHT, E. O. (1979) *Class, Crisis and the State*, London, Verso.

WRIGHT, N. (1989) *Assessing Radical Education: A Critical Review of the Radical Movement in English Schooling, 1960–1980*, Milton Keynes, Open University Press.

WOODROOFE, K. (1962) *From Charity to Social Work*, London, Routledge and Kegan Paul.

YOUNG, M. F. D. (Ed.) (1971) *Knowledge and Control*, London, Macmillan.

YOUNG, M. and WHITTY, G. (1977) 'Introduction: Perspectives on education and society', in YOUNG, M. and WHITTY, G. (Eds) *Society, State and Schooling*, London, Falmer Press.

YOUNG, M. and WILLMOTT, P. (1962) *Family and Kinship in East London*, Harmondsworth, Penguin.

ZARETSKY, E. (1976) *Capitalism: The Family and Personal Life*, London, Pluto Press.

ZARETSKY, E. (1982) 'The place of the family in the origins of the welfare state', in THORNE, B. and YALLOM, M. (Eds) *Rethinking the Family: Some Feminist Questions*, Harlow, Longman.

Index